LOW-CARB COOKBOOK

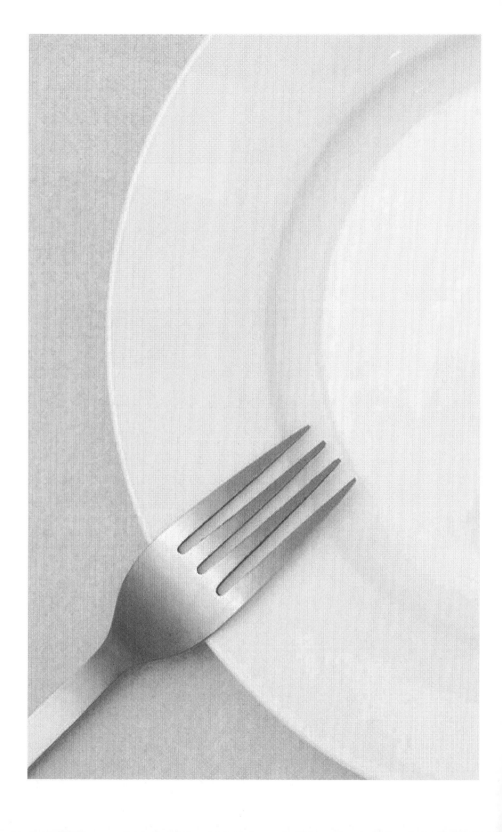

Low-Carb Cookbook

125 Easy, Healthy, and Delicious
Recipes for a Low-Carb Diet

MENDOCINO PRESS

Contents

14-Day Meal Plan

Breakfast

Snacks and Appetizers

CHAPTER EIGHT

Soups and Stews   69

CHAPTER NINE

Salads 91

CHAPTER TEN

Side Dishes 109

CHAPTER ELEVEN

Vegetarian Entrées 121

CHAPTER TWELVE

Fish and Seafood 135

Poultry, Pork, and Beef 149

Desserts 169

Introduction

C hances are you've heard all about low-carb diets: Hollywood celebrities credit their amazing bodies to it, and talk shows and magazines tout it as the quick-fix solution to low energy and weight gain. Well, there's a reason it gets so much publicity: It works! A low-carb diet can help you lose weight, improve your cholesterol, and reduce your risk of heart disease, diabetes, high blood pressure, and cardiovascular disease. On top of that, low-carb diets may also help improve your energy, mood, and ability to concentrate. Who *wouldn't* want all those things?

There's more good news: While other diets may leave you bored with limited choices, starving over tiny portion sizes, and cranky over cardboard-tasting dishes, a low-carb diet doesn't. You still get to eat delicious, flavor-packed foods and enjoy all your favorite dishes—you just need to make a few important adjustments. That's where this book will help you. In the first half of the book, you'll learn what a low-carb diet really means (hint: it's more than just tossing your pasta and bread into the trash), why you should try it, what health benefits you can expect, and how to make the transition as seamlessly as possible. Along the way, this book will teach you the following:

- Easy tips on how to reduce your consumption of carbs

- How to spot which seemingly innocent foods and drinks actually hide a ton of carbs

- Simple cooking tips and ingredient substitutions to make any dish low-carb

- What to buy at the grocery store so you can stock up on healthful, low-carb foods

- How to stick to your low-carb diet when dining out

You'll also get a detailed, 14-day meal plan that takes the guesswork out of adopting a low-carb diet so you can get started right away.

Once you understand the basics, it's time to get cooking! The second half of this book is packed with 125 tasty, easy, and quick low-carb recipes that won't leave you wondering where the flavor went. The best part? All your favorite comfort foods are included. You'll find recipes for these tasty meals and more:

- Breakfast, such as Baked Eggs in Ham Cups (page 45) and Turkey and Apple Breakfast Sausage (page 50)

- Snacks and appetizers, such as Hot and Smoky Nuts (page 54) and Chicken Skewers with Tomato, Lemon, and Rosemary (page 62)

- Soups and stews, such as Broccoli Cheddar Soup (page 77) and Jambalaya (page 90)

- Salads, such as Caesar Salad with Mushrooms (page 98) and Spicy Shrimp and Black Bean Salad (page 105)

- Side dishes, such as Classic Coleslaw with a Spicy Twist (page 113) and Stuffing with Sausage and Herbs (page 120)

- Vegetarian entrées, such as Eggplant Parmesan (page 129) and Spaghetti Squash Alfredo (page 132)

- Fish and seafood, such as Fish Tacos with Mango Salsa (page 143) and Brown Sugar and Mustard Grilled Salmon (page 147)

- Poultry, pork, and beef, such as Chicken Paprikash (page 153), Slow Cooker Roast Pork Shoulder with German Spices (page 161), and Skirt Steak with Garlic-Herb Sauce (page 166)

- Desserts, such as Almond Cheesecake Bars (page 186) and Chocolate Truffles (page 185)

Getting hungry? What are you waiting for?! Read on to learn how you can adopt a low-carb diet and whip up some delicious dishes that will leave you feeling healthy and happy about the changes you've made.

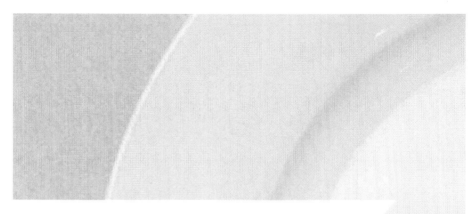

CHAPTER ONE

Why Choose a Low-Carb Diet?

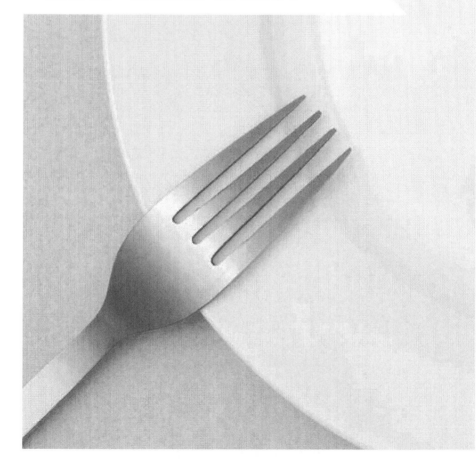

Why Choose a Low-Carb Diet?

For anyone who wants to improve his or her health, there are seemingly limitless options out there: South Beach, Atkins, Mediterranean, raw food, and gluten-free diets all vie for your attention. You can cut out all meat, live solely on meat, go fat-free, boost your fat intake—it's enough to make you hit the drive-through. But before you do, take some time to learn about eating low-carb. Unlike fad diets, a low-carb diet is a natural way of eating that improves much more than the number you see on the scale (although, yes, it will do that, too).

What Are Carbohydrates?

To understand what a low-carb diet is, you first have to know what a carbohydrate is. This little bit of Nutrition 101 will help the diet make sense to you.

Basically, all the food you eat is made up of three macronutrients: fats, proteins, and carbohydrates. Fats and proteins are pretty easily identified: foods like butter and oil are fats; meat, fish, legumes, and eggs contain protein. While it is important to watch our intake of fats, our bodies require a certain amount to function properly; fats store energy and help proteins do their jobs. Protein gives you energy, carries nutrients, helps the immune function, helps grow and repair cells, and keeps the brain running smoothly. Carbohydrates, however, can be tougher to spot because they occur in many different types of foods—fruits, vegetables, grains (breads and cereals), dairy products, and sugar. Your body uses carbohydrates to create glucose (a.k.a. blood sugar), which in turn gives you energy and fuels your brain and nervous system. Sounds pretty good, right?

It's a little more complicated than that. Within the broad category of carbohydrates, there are two main types: simple and complex. Simple carbohydrates are generally classified as refined sugars that don't deliver many nutrients but can be high in calories. They are also broken down quickly by your body, resulting in a rush of energy followed by a crash (sound familiar?). Foods containing simple carbohydrates include the following:

- Candy

- Cereal

- Fruit

- Sugar

- Jam and jelly

- Juice

- Milk and milk products

- Soda

- White flour

Milk products and fruit do contain some nutrients. But white flour, sugar, soda, and candy provide mostly empty calories.

On the other hand, complex carbohydrates have a more, well, complex structure and are usually rich in fiber, vitamins, and minerals. Because of this, your body takes longer to digest complex carbohydrates, which makes them a great, long-lasting source of energy. Whenever possible, choose complex carbohydrates over simple ones to help even out your energy levels and contribute to weight loss.

Foods with complex carbohydrates include the following:

- Whole-grain bread

- Oatmeal

- Spinach

- Sweet potatoes

- Beans and lentils

Now that you know what a carbohydrate is, it's time to learn what qualifies as a low-carbohydrate diet.

Fiber is a complex carbohydrate that is healthful for your heart and occurs naturally in a lot of different foods. For every 1,000 calories you consume, aim for 14 grams of dietary fiber (28 grams in a 2,000-calorie diet). To increase how much fiber you eat, up your consumption of beans, whole grains, whole fruits, and vegetables.

What Is a Low-Carb Diet?

In its simplest form, a low-carb diet is exactly what it sounds like: You cut down on the total amount of carbohydrates you consume (both simple and complex). In other words, you substantially reduce your intake of items like breads, pastas, and starchy vegetables.

Why? It isn't that eating carbohydrates is bad; it's simply that most people eat way more carbohydrates than they need to keep their bodies humming along. When you eat too many carbohydrates—more than your body can use for immediate energy—your body stores them for later use or converts them to fat. A moment on the lips really can mean a lifetime on the hips (or upper arms or butt) when it comes to too many carbs. But the opposite also holds true: Cut down on carbohydrates, and your body will start to use the fat you have stored around your body for energy, resulting in weight loss and a trimmer physique.

By adopting a low-carb diet, you will find yourself eating more protein and fat during snacks and meals. That means instead of having noodles or breads as the main component, you'll have more fish, meat, eggs, and low-carb vegetables as the base. This increases the vitamins and nutrients you're consuming—another benefit of a low-carb diet (more on that soon).

Under the umbrella of low-carb diets, many different brand-name diets exist: The Atkins Diet, South Beach Diet, Sugar Busters Diet, and Paleo Diet are all, at their core, low-carb diets.

The **Atkins Diet** has four different phases, including the super-restrictive beginning phase when you aren't allowed to eat a single piece of fruit or bread for 2 weeks. You are gradually allowed to add carbohydrates back in via fibrous vegetables. It is generally known as a very strict diet.

The **South Beach Diet**, like Atkins, also has different phases, but focuses on the glycemic index (GI) of different foods. You're allowed some carbohydrates, but only the ones that are low on the index. It also emphasizes small portion sizes and eating only until your hunger goes away—concepts that are important to anyone hoping to lose weight.

> **The glycemic index (GI) is a way of categorizing how fast your blood sugar rises after eating a specific food.** The simple carbs that break down quickly in the body have a higher GI level, while complex carbs that take a longer time to digest have a lower GI. Sticking to low-GI foods is another way of avoiding simple carbs.

The **Sugar Busters Diet** shines a spotlight on refined sugar—a simple carbohydrate—and how overindulging in it leads to weight gain. In a nutshell, you aren't allowed to eat any refined sugars, including corn syrup, molasses, and honey. On this diet, you are allowed only around 1,200 calories a day—such a small amount of food that you are practically guaranteed to lose weight (if you can stick with it).

While some low-carb diets have been around for decades, the hottest diet trend right now has actually been around for *thousands* of years. The **Paleo Diet** asks us to eat like our ancestors, the cavemen, ate. Anything that wasn't around 10,000 years ago is out, including carbohydrates like dairy, grains, legumes, and refined sugars.

While all these diets have unique guidelines and eating plans, the one thing they share is an emphasis on cutting back carbohydrates.

What Are the Health Benefits of a Low-Carb Diet?

Now that you understand the basics of a low-carb diet, you're probably wondering about the health benefits of the program and why you should give it a shot. You don't have to be a nutritionist to realize that replacing pizza and lasagna with chicken and salads is going to improve your health, but there's more to it than that.

The biggest benefit to lowering your intake of carbohydrates is weight loss. When you aren't overeating carbs, your body will begin to use stored fat for energy, helping you slim down and stay that way. Dieters who go low-carb have been found to have higher resting metabolisms (the amount of calories you burn at rest), which helps to explain why they don't just lose weight but keep it off in the long term.

You'll also find that you won't need to eat as much on a low-carb diet. All the protein and fat you're digesting will keep you feeling full longer. In other words, you're going to avoid that afternoon crash that has you crawling to the vending machine for a quick shot of candy. With longer digestion times, you won't get as hungry between meals and snacks. That's why low-carb diets don't feel like other diets. You aren't restricting amounts of food and starving yourself to see a difference in how your jeans fit. You're just making better choices every time you eat.

The combination of weight loss, which benefits your body in countless ways, and the increased consumption of more healthful, nutrient-rich complex carbs has many positive effects: You may also reduce your risk for diabetes (fewer carbs in your diet mean lower levels of blood sugar), high blood pressure, stroke, cardiovascular disease, high cholesterol, and other serious health issues.

Because obesity is such a big issue in America today, researchers continue to study the effects of different diets on weight. When they examine low-carb diets, the findings are encouraging. In fact, a recent review of studies showed that obese participants on a low-carb diet lost weight while improving their waist circumference, blood pressure, triglycerides, blood sugar, heart disease risk factors, and cholesterol levels.

In addition to physical improvements, there are some commonly reported mental health benefits to following a low-carb diet, including a noticeable improvement in energy levels. Since low-carb foods take longer to digest than simple sugars, the energy boost experienced after meals and snacks is prolonged. Increased energy is often accompanied by a better mood and general feeling of well-being (plus better sleep patterns at night). Some people also notice that they don't crave sweets as much as they used to. Once your body goes through detox and gets used to the small amount of sugar you're eating, you'll be satisfied with a lot less of it. Even a piece of fresh fruit will taste like candy!

When you switch to a low-carb diet, the amount of processed sugar you eat is drastically reduced. You have to be a lot more selective about what you eat, cutting way back on sugar-filled sodas, candy, cookies, cakes, and cereals. One surprising benefit is healthier teeth: When sugar constantly hangs out in your mouth, you have a higher risk for cavities and gum disease. Nix the colas, super-sweet salad dressings, and hard candy, for example, and your dental hygiene improves drastically.

Cutting out carbs can also improve the health of people who may not realize they have a gluten sensitivity (gluten is found in carbohydrates such as wheat and other grains). Unlike celiac disease or wheat allergies, which can be quite extreme, a gluten sensitivity results in bloating, diarrhea, bone or joint pain, headaches, and other issues. By adopting a low-carb diet, you automatically reduce your intake of gluten-containing foods, which could lessen any of these symptoms.

Make a simple decision to lower your carbohydrate consumption, and you'll discover the key to looking and feeling better than ever. You could lose weight, feel more energized, lower your risk for serious health issues, improve your dental hygiene, feel less bloated, and sleep better. By becoming more aware of what you put into your body and how those eating choices affect you, you are well on your way to becoming the healthiest, happiest version of yourself.

CHAPTER TWO

Getting Started on a Low-Carb Diet

It's one thing to decide to follow a low-carb diet but quite another to actually do it. In this chapter, you'll get all the practical information necessary to get started.

Tips for Sucessfully Adopting a Low-Carb Diet

A lot of information is swirling around about how to follow a low-carb diet. Some is true; some not so much. Let's start with the basics: To follow a low-carb diet, you need to reduce the amount of carbohydrates you eat. This means becoming aware of what foods have carbs lurking in them and how much (see chapter 3).

Remove the Temptations. Before kicking off your low-carb eating plan, go through your kitchen—refrigerator and pantry—and toss or donate food that will tempt you to go back to your old ways: sugary processed treats, white rice, sweetened drinks, crackers, and chips. You will be much likelier to stick to your game plan if you have only healthful options at home.

Become a Picky Eater. You also need to become pickier about what type of carbohydrates you eat. You can successfully eat a low-carb diet while still filling up on junk food and soft drinks. This isn't the way to go. Remember this rule: Choose complex over simple carbs whenever possible to get the best fuel for your body. Just because you're allowed a certain amount of carbohydrates every day doesn't mean you should get it from nutritionless fare.

So what are the best choices for carbohydrates? Whole grains such as whole wheat, brown rice, bulgur, quinoa, and wild rice as well as legumes such as lentils, black beans, chickpeas, kidney beans, and soybeans. All of these will give you nutritional bang for your buck and fill you up, and they won't spike your blood sugar or lead to a quick energy crash.

Keep a Food Journal. Cutting back doesn't mean cutting out—that's an important distinction. The goal here is not to stop eating all carbohydrates (as you've learned, you need some carbs to get energy and help your body function properly). The goal is to eat less of them. One way to do this is to start keeping a food journal or log. Whenever you eat something, jot down what it is and how many carbohydrates are in it. You can find this information on the food label or online (more on this in chapter 4). This way, you'll be able to calculate your total carbohydrate intake day in and day out. Once you get into this practice and learn how many carbs the foods you eat contain, you won't need to keep up with the food diary. But in the beginning it will be really helpful to your success.

Studies have shown that people who keep a food journal lose more weight than those who don't. If you really want to keep a detailed account, include the time of day and how you're feeling at the time you eat. This approach will help you notice emotional eating patterns and pinpoint when you seem to lose the willpower to stick with your goal.

Daily Carb Guidelines

Let's get to the nitty-gritty of low-carb diets and how many carbohydrates you should consume in a day.

Typical Recommendations

The Recommended Daily Intake (RDI) of carbs varies quite a bit depending on what source you read. Here's how many grams of carbohydrate three different organizations recommend the average American should consume on a 2,000-calorie-a-day diet (not someone following a low-carb diet):

U.S. Department of Agriculture (USDA): 225 grams a day

Food and Drug Administration (FDA): 300 grams a day

Institute of Medicine (IOM): 130 grams per day

So what number should you aim for if you want to follow a low-carb diet? Again, that's up for debate. Some diets want you to start by consuming as low as 20 grams of carbohydrates in a day, but that's an incredibly low number that's hard to reach or sustain. Other low-carb diets recommend you consume 50 grams a day or, if you're physically active, up to 100 grams a day. That said, most experts agree that 100 to 150 grams of carbs a day is a relatively good, low-carb target. You'll need to see what works best for you and personalize your daily intake (low enough to see weight loss but high enough that you have energy and aren't starving).

Let's say you're aiming for 75 grams of carbohydrates a day. If you eat three meals and two snacks a day, that might be 15 to 20 grams of carbohydrates per meal and 5 to 10 grams of carbs per snack. That's not a lot! That's why it's important to learn how many carbs are in your favorite foods and keep a food journal so you can jot down your intake as you go along. Fortunately, we have some tips to help keep you on track.

10 Tips to Reduce Your Consumption of Carbs

1. **Pay more attention to what you're eating.** You've probably spent most of your life eating high-carb foods without really noticing. It's not your fault! The food and restaurant industries have made it super easy to fill up our plates with carbs. Think about it: The rolls in the basket at restaurants, the sandwich bread surrounding your favorite turkey club, the pasta in the salad bar—carbohydrates are lurking everywhere. If you don't focus on what you're putting into your body, you'll ruin any low-carb plans you may have. So every time you're about to eat, take a moment to figure out what foods on the table are packed with carbohydrates. Choose one carbohydrate to eat and stop there. If you really want the dinner roll, then go ahead and eat it but realize you can't also have pasta or potatoes with your entrée. In time, you'll be able to quickly decide which carb is worth it to you and which you can skip without a care.

2. **Become a portion minimizer.** You don't want to go through life saying no to every carbohydrate-heavy dish you're offered. Instead, say yes but serve yourself only a small portion. Portion control is probably going

to be a big shift for you. A serving size of pasta is ½ cup, not the 2 cups that fill up a plate or bowl. Measure it out (you won't have to every time; just until you recognize what a portion looks like) and stick to that amount. You could also try out these tips to reduce portion size: Instead of a normal-size piece of cake or pie, get just a sliver; instead of the club sandwich, order a regular one and eat it open-faced with only one slice of bread; instead of the super-size fries, get a kid-size order and split it with a friend. Eventually, a few bites of whatever food you want will be enough to cure your craving without affecting your weight loss goals or how you feel.

Remembering how big a portion should be can help you lose weight faster. There are different tricks you can use the next time you're serving yourself: ½ cup is about half the size of a baseball, a bagel should be only the size of a can of tuna, and a slice of bread should be about the size of a CD case.

3. **Cut out all processed food.** This is really something everybody should be doing, but it's especially important for those who are trying to follow a low-carb diet. Most snack foods and packaged foods are full of carbohydrates and sugar (another carbohydrate, not to mention empty calories) and are low in vitamins, nutrients, and fiber. These include crackers, cookies, cereals, snack cakes, granola bars, and candy, to name just a few.

4. **Stay away from starches.** It can be tough to remember what veggies are on the "avoid" list when you're eating low-carb. A great rule of thumb is to consider if the vegetable is starchy. Potatoes and corn, for example, are super starchy and also high in carbohydrates. Kale, mushrooms, avocado, and spinach, on the other hand, aren't starchy and are great options.

5. **Stop being afraid of fat.** In the 1980s, fat-free diets were very popular. People would eat as much as they wanted, as long as it was low-fat. Unfortunately, low-fat items are often high in sugar and calories to make up for the flavor that is lost when the fat is taken away. That fad diet quickly lost its popularity when people noticed they weren't actually losing weight and how horrible everything tasted. So now it's time to realize that fat can be your friend. Fat can help you feel full and satisfied after a meal—like you've really treated yourself. That being

said, saturated fats—those found in red meat and dairy products like butter—aren't the best idea. However, there are many great sources of heart-healthful unsaturated fats: Think nuts, extra-virgin olive oil, avocado, and salmon. A lot of the recipes in this book embrace healthful fats and so should you.

6. **Pack protein in whenever you can.** You are going to be cutting down on carbs, so to replace those foods you should be eating a lot more protein. Protein is hard to overeat, maintains a high energy level for a long time, and is delicious! Every time you plan a meal or snack, start by deciding on your protein. Breakfast should include eggs or some kind of meat; lunch and dinner should focus on fish, poultry, or beef; and between-meal snacks should include nuts or a high-protein dairy to boost your intake.

7. **Make some simple swaps.** Many traditionally carb-centric dishes can be made in a lighter way but will still retain their flavor. Turn burrito night into lettuce-wrap night. Enjoy your homemade tomato sauce over spaghetti squash instead of spaghetti noodles. And whenever you have the option, swap out white carbs for whole grains—whole-wheat bread, whole-wheat pasta, and brown rice. Many low-carb diets suggest thinking of it as a "no white diet": Many things that are white—potatoes, rice, sugar, flour—should be cut out. (See the handy substitution chart in chapter 3, page 18).

8. **Rethink the ratio on your plate.** Most people begin meals by loading their plate with the carb first: the mashed potatoes or pasta or rice that will go under anything else you're eating. Instead, first load up three-quarters of your plate with veggies and protein, then, in the quarter that's left over, serve yourself a small portion of the carbohydrate. It's different than how you've done it before, but it will help keep carbs to a minimum while upping your intake of the good stuff.

9. **Drink only water or other simple beverages.** So many drinks are high in calories, sugar, and carbohydrates. Think about it: Sodas, juices, café mochas, smoothies, sports drinks, bottled iced teas, and lemonade are all crammed with more sugar than you can shake a teaspoon at. By drinking anything besides simple water or tea or coffee, you are sabotaging yourself and making it almost impossible to lower your carb intake. If you need more flavor, try infusing your water with fruit or cucumber. Or go with seltzer—the bubbles make it seem more fun than straight-from-the-tap water and give you the sense that you're treating

yourself. You can even make your own iced tea without any added sugar and keep a pitcher in the fridge to reach for whenever you're craving it.

10. **Allow yourself a cheat every now and then.** Go ahead and occasionally cheat, to satisfy that nagging craving. But the keys to cheating is that you don't do it too often, you choose smartly, you have a sensibly small portion, and you savor every single bite. You aren't allowed to cheat and have a big bowl of ice cream every night. But, if you happen to be on vacation and walk by an ice-cream shop with incredible premium flavors, get a small kid-size scoop, sit down, and slowly relish each spoonful (but skip the sugar cone). With this approach, you won't feel guilty afterward because you know you're allowed to indulge on occasion without undoing all your hard work.

CHAPTER THREE

Identifying High- and Low-Carb Foods

It's almost impossible to eat a low-carb diet if you have no idea which foods are high in carbs and which are low—and it's not quite as easy to tell the difference as you might imagine. Some foods you'd think would get the green light are actually best avoided, and vice versa. In this chapter, you'll learn where your favorite foods fall on the carb spectrum, which will help you make better choices.

Everyday Foods and Beverages High in Carbs

Consider this the "avoid whenever possible" section. These foods and beverages are fine in small portions as part of a dish (and some offer essential nutrients, fiber, and vitamins), but don't create an entire meal out of them.

1. **Grains.** When most people hear the word *carbohydrate,* they think grains. That's for good reason. One slice of bread has around 14 grams of carbs (which means that when you slap two slices down on a plate to make a sandwich, you're already hitting 28 grams). It's tough to find bread items that aren't carb bombs. Just ate a bagel? You've downed up to 60 grams of carbs (without cream cheese or jam spread on top). Want some cereal? One cup of Shredded Wheat has 39 grams of carbs. One cup of Cheerios contains 20 grams of carbs. Muffins, pancakes, hamburger buns, and croissants are all similarly high in carbs. If you do eat a bread item, and you will from time to time, always opt for something made with whole grains to get as much fiber as possible. And remember that something doesn't have to be a bread product to be

made from grain. Flour comes from wheat, so anything made with flour, such as pasta and pizza dough, is also high in carbs. Also watch out for grains other than wheat, like rice (1 cup has 45 grams of carbs), barley (1 cup has 135 grams of carbs), and oats (1 cup has 103 grams of carbs).

2. **Sweetened foods.** Granulated sugar (you know, the kind you stir into coffee or mix into cookie batter) is 100 percent carbohydrates. The more sugary the thing is that you're putting in your mouth, the greater the carb load it carries. The worst of the worst are hard candies and gummy candies: They're made almost entirely from sugar, which means they're almost pure carbohydrates. But all other sweets—candies, cakes, puddings, and cookies—get a red flag as well. You can still have them every now and then (come on, this is life after all), but they need to be something you rarely splurge on as opposed to being something you indulge in once a day (or more often).

3. **Drinks.** It's not just what you eat that you need to mind. Drinks can be just as potent a source of carbs, sometimes even more so. Just 1 cup of Gatorade (and who has only 1 cup?) has 15 grams of carbs; 1 cup of orange juice has 30 grams; and a can of soda has 39 grams. Go for a fountain soft drink and you're looking at 45 grams of carbs or more! And don't forget about booze. While it's totally fine to have an alcoholic drink every now and then, imbibing too often can ruin your low-carb goals. Sweet wines can contain a lot of carbs from the grapes; mixers like sodas and juices are typically carb-laden; and beers are made out of grains and may contain up to 20 grams of carbs per can (12 fluid ounces).

As opposed to regular sodas, diet sodas contain almost no carbs because they use artificial sweeteners. That said, researchers and nutritionists are torn on whether or not diet soda is a smart choice nutritionally. Some studies have shown that even people who drink diet sodas are more likely to be overweight than those who skip soda altogether.

4. **Starchy vegetables.** A little less obvious but just as important to watch are starchy vegetables. Remember, starches are complex carbohydrates that our bodies turn into sugar during digestion. A baked potato, without a single topping, can have as much as 49 grams of carbs per serving. French fries, hash browns, potato chips—all are made up almost

exclusively of potatoes and all are packing tons of carbohydrates. Other starchy vegetables you should limit include sweet potatoes, yams, corn (1 cup of kernels has 36 grams of carbs), peas, and all the different kinds of squash like acorn and butternut. Compared to potatoes, however, squash has fewer carbs, so if you had to pick one from this list, go with the squash (plus you'll get lots of great nutrients from the squash).

5. **Fruit.** Because of the load of natural sugars they contain, fruit includes some big carb offenders. The sweetest varieties—dates (one has 18 grams of carbs), cherries (1 cup has 12.5 grams of carbs), grapes (1 cup has 27 grams of carbs), mangoes (1 cup has almost 25 grams of carbs), pears (one has 27 grams of carbs), and pineapple (1 cup has 21 grams of carbs)—are also the worst for someone on a low-carb diet. Watch out, too, for bananas, which can be as starchy and carb-laden as a potato: A medium banana can have as much as 27 grams. Be even more careful when it comes to dried fruit; the concentrated sugars and ease of bingeing due to their small size make raisins and other dried fruits super-high-carb items.

Sneaky Carbs

Now that we've reviewed which obvious foods and drinks are high in carbohydrates, it's time to discover some surprising places carbs are lurking.

1. **Cooked beans.** While these are often thought of as being high in protein, they are also high in carbohydrates: 1 cup of great Northern beans clocks in at 37 grams of carbs; 1 cup of black beans has 40 grams; 1 cup of cannellini has 46 grams; and 1 cup of lentils is up there at 40 grams.

2. **Dairy products.** It's natural for most people to hear *dairy* and think protein and calcium, but milk also has a lot of naturally occurring sugars that lead to a high carbohydrate count. While different types of milk (whole versus skim) have slightly different carb loads, a good rule of thumb is that 1 cup of milk has about 11.5 grams of carbohydrates. Dairy products such as yogurt also have a bit of carbs, but it's often the added sugar that's the bigger culprit.

3. **Low-fat foods.** Low-fat products are often billed as health foods, but surprisingly they are often high-carb items. When companies remove the fat from processed fare like muffins, cookies, and crackers, they typically add loads of sugar to make the end product taste better. If

you're going to eat something high in carbs, go with the full-fat version and you'll at least feel satisfied afterward.

4. **Sauces and dressings.** Most of these, like barbecue sauce, bottled salad dressings, marinades, and ketchup, are loaded with sugar and high-fructose corn syrup and, therefore, loaded with carbs.

Low-Carb Foods and Beverages

Now some good news: While it seems as if there are a lot of foods high in carbohydrates, there are just as many that are low in carbohydrates. Anybody taking on a low-carb diet has loads of options. Focus on what you can have instead of what you can't, and you'll never have bored taste buds.

1. **Meat and seafood.** This is probably the biggest category of low-carb foods. Beef, chicken, pork, and seafood are so high in protein, with a little fat mixed in, that there's little room for carbs. Just watch out how you prepare them. *Do* grill, bake, and roast. *Don't* bread them (like fried chicken) or dunk them in sugary sauces like honey mustard or barbecue sauce. Also keep in mind that processed deli meats like ham, hot dogs, and sausages might have added sugar in them, so check the nutrition label.

2. **Nonstarchy vegetables.** Eat as many nonstarchy vegetables as you'd like! The list includes all kinds of greens (lettuces, spinach, chard, kale, radicchio, endive, etc.), sprouts, celery, radishes, mushrooms, avocado, asparagus, cucumbers, green beans, fennel, cauliflower, broccoli, peppers, squash (in moderation), Brussels sprouts, tomatoes, artichokes, and herbs. You have tons of options, so there's no need to feel stuck in a veggie rut.

3. **Nuts and seeds.** Lower in carbs, nuts and seeds are good for snacking (just watch your portion size—you should limit yourself to a small handful because they are high in fat), at mealtime (nut butters are delicious), and baking (some nuts can be turned into flour). A 1-ounce handful of almonds has only 2.7 grams of carbs; 1 ounce hazelnuts has 4.7 grams; 1 ounce macadamia nuts, 4 grams; 1 ounce peanuts, 4.5 grams; and 1 ounce pecans, 3.9 grams. To top it off, nuts are super filling and contain heart-healthful unsaturated fats.

4. **Lower-carb beverage options.** When it comes to beverages, things get a little trickier. You aren't stuck with just water and club soda (although,

honestly, plain water should make up the majority of your beverage consumption). If you want iced tea, make it yourself and don't add any sugar (throw in some fresh mint leaves while it's cooling and you'll get the flavor boost you crave). You can also go sugar-free with drink mixes such as the kind made by Crystal Light. Coffee and hot tea drinkers can rejoice! As long as you don't dump loads of sugar or honey into your drink or sip on something like a mocha, you are free and clear to enjoy. As for alcohol, if you're choosing wine, go with red since it's packed with antioxidants and has only 3 to 5 grams of carbs per 100-gram glass (white wine has the same carb amount, there are just fewer studies showing its health benefits). If you like to sip on a little whiskey every now and then or mix scotch with some club soda, you can relax knowing that pure liquor is actually carb-free—it's the mixers you need to worry about.

Many studies have shown health benefits to having one alcoholic drink a day. Drinking alcohol in moderation can reduce your risk of developing heart disease, stroke, gallstones, and diabetes. The key is to stick to one glass a day (and no, that doesn't mean you can abstain all week and have seven drinks on Saturday night).

Low-Carb Substitutes

One of the smartest strategies for sticking to a low-carb diet is to have some go-to substitutions. That way you can enjoy your favorite dishes with a few swaps and still hit your carbohydrate goal for the day. Just use this handy chart and you'll keep your stomach happy *and* your abs flat.

Low-Carb Substitutions

Instead of ...	Use ...
Milk, 2% (11.5 grams of carbs per 1 cup)	✓ Unsweetened soy milk (2 to 5 grams of carbs per 1 cup)
White flour (95 grams of carbs per 1 cup)	✓ Almond flour (8 grams of carbs per 1 cup) ✓ Coconut flour (80 grams of carbs per 1 cup, but extremely high in fiber) ✓ Flaxseed meal (20 grams of carbs per 1 cup) (Unfortunately, you can't just swap them one for one in your regular recipe, but there are tons of resources out there for baked goods using low-carb alternatives.)
White sandwich bread (12 grams of carbs per slice)	✓ Low-carb tortillas (they're packed with so much fiber, the net carb count is only 3 to 6 grams per tortilla) ✓ Lettuce wraps (cut the carbs down to almost nothing)
Pasta (43 grams of carbs per 1 cup of spaghetti)	✓ Spaghetti squash (see recipe, page 132; 7 grams of carbs per 1 cup) ✓ Zucchini (thinly slice and layer in place of lasagna noodles)
Potatoes (35 grams of carbs per 1 medium potato; 17 grams of carbs per ½ cup of mashed potatoes)	✓ Cauliflower (1.5 grams of carbs per ½ cup; can be mashed, shredded and turned into hash browns, or even cut up to fake spuds in potato salad)

CHAPTER FOUR

Shopping, Cooking, and Eating Low-Carb

What good is knowledge if you can't translate it to real life? Now that you know what foods are high in carbs and which aren't, it's time to head to the grocery store, kitchen, and restaurant. This chapter provides tips for tackling grocery shopping and cooking low-carb, and includes a tip list for keeping you on track when dining out.

Shopping Tips

Want to be a low-carb supermarket star? Avoid the bread aisle or the bakery—especially if you're just starting on your low-carb journey and are still in the "I miss bread" zone. You might begin your shopping trip with the best intentions, but seeing all those freshly baked loaves could push your willpower to its limit. So do yourself a favor and don't even go there.

While we're at it, avoid the center aisles in the grocery store, too. Most of the food found down those aisles (high-carb, highly processed snacks, meals, beverages, and desserts) really aren't your friends either. It's best to avoid them.

You've probably heard it before, but shopping the perimeter of the grocery store is the best way to fill your cart with healthful food. Fruits, vegetables, meat, and dairy can usually all be found without a single turn down an aisle. Fill your cart with those foods.

There is one aisle, however, that you *will* want to go down: the frozen-food aisle. Stock up on frozen fruits and veggies (*not* French fries) to make throwing together a last-minute meal as easy as possible.

Frozen produce may be even better for you than some of the fresh varieties. Freshly picked produce are frozen right when those fruits and vegetables are at their peak—meaning they have more nutrients than at any other time. The stuff in the produce aisle might have been picked before reaching ripeness and can be many days old, so the concentration of nutrients could be lower.

Just because you're going low-carb doesn't mean you have to be high-cost. Box stores like Sam's Club sell staples in bulk, which can lower your ultimate grocery bill by hundreds of dollars. Stock up on meat, long-lasting produce like onions, and pantry items like chicken broth. Then head to the grocery store or farmers' market for perishable items or things you need in smaller quantities.

Low-Carb Shopping List. Here's how to make grocery shopping as simple as possible: Focus on buying items on this list. It's not exhaustive—spices, for example, aren't on it—but it's a great place to start and will keep you low-carb focused.

Meat

Bacon	Pork chops
Beef	Pork tenderloin
Chicken	Pot roast
Ground beef and turkey	Sausage
Ham	Turkey

Seafood

Crab	Scallops
Halibut	Shrimp
Salmon	Tuna steaks

Dairy

Butter	Eggs
Cheddar cheese	Greek yogurt, plain
Cream	Parmesan cheese
Cream cheese	Sour cream (low-fat)

Produce

Artichokes	Garlic
Asparagus	Green beans
Avocados	Green onions
Bell peppers	Kale
Berries	Leeks
Bok choy	Lettuce
Broccoli	Mushrooms
Brussels sprouts	Onions
Cabbage	Peas (in moderation)
Cauliflower	Rhubarb
Celery	Spinach
Cucumbers	Squash (in moderation)

Other foods

Almond flour	Mayonnaise (light)
Almonds	Peanut butter or almond butter
Beef jerky	Pecans
Canned tuna	Sesame oil
Crushed tomatoes	Soy sauce (reduced-sodium)
Dijon mustard	Sun-dried tomatoes
Extra-virgin olive oil	Walnuts
Hazelnuts	

How to Read Food Labels. With so many items on grocery store shelves to choose from, it can be a little daunting figuring out what to buy. How can you tell which items are best for you? Turn the package around and examine the food label. You can have the best intentions, but to eat healthfully and successfully follow a low-carb diet, you need to be able to determine which foods to leave on the shelf.

You might assume that the total carbohydrates listed on a food label will tell you everything you need to know—unfortunately, this isn't the case. Keep scanning and also look for the amount of fiber per serving. Although fiber is a form of carbohydrate (it's included in the total carb count), your body has a tough time converting fiber to glucose (sugar), and sometimes it can't convert it at all. As a result, carbs from fiber don't have the same consequences in your body as regular carbohydrates, which means the amount of dietary fiber can be subtracted from the total carbohydrate amount to give you your net carb total. For example, let's say a package of soup has 15 grams of carbohydrates and 4 grams of fiber. The net carbs are only 9 grams—that's a big improvement!

While you won't find net carbs listed on food labels, you will find it listed in the recipes in this book. In fact, every recipe includes two carb counts: gross and net. Gross carbohydrates include everything, while net takes out the carbs that come from fiber.

Cooking Tips

Low-carb cooking doesn't differ all that much from regular cooking—you are still baking, sautéing, roasting, boiling, and steaming. But there are a few small areas where you may need to make some adjustments.

Cooking Meat and Seafood. When eating low-carb, beef, chicken, pork, and seafood usually take a front-and-center role in meals, so if you aren't comfortable cooking them, you should get there. The most important thing to remember is that if the meat is ground (such as ground beef or turkey, or sausage), it needs to be cooked all the way through (the grinding process can incorporate bacteria throughout). Chicken also needs to be cooked completely (to avoid salmonella poisoning). Other meats, like beef, pork, and fish, can be cooked less depending on personal taste.

You can make the whole process a lot easier by buying an instant-read thermometer and checking the thickest part of the meat to see if it meets the minimum cooking temperature guidelines. Otherwise you have to cut into it to test for doneness, which can cause juices to flow out and your meat to taste dry. (Most chefs recommend letting meat sit for 10 minutes after you finish cooking it to let the juices evenly distribute themselves again.)

Minimum Cooking Temperatures for Meat and Seafood

Beef, veal, and lamb:
Medium-rare: 120 to 130°F
Well-done: 170°F

Ground beef: 160°F

Pork:
Medium: 160°F
Well-done: 170°F

Ground pork: 160°F

Poultry (chicken and turkey, including ground): 165°F

Seafood:
>Fish: 145°F or until flesh is opaque and flakes easily with a fork
>Shrimp, crab, lobster: Cook until flesh is pearly and opaque
>Scallops: Cook until flesh is opaque and firm
>Clams, mussels, and oysters: Cook until shells open; discard any
>>that remain closed after cooking

When cooking fish, you don't have to be as specific about temperature. To see if your fish is fully cooked, take the back of a spoon and press it against the flesh of the fillet—it should just begin to flake. Fish will continue cooking for a few minutes after you take it off the heat, so don't overcook it, or you'll end up with a dry dinner. When it comes to tuna and salmon, you can cook it so the inside is a little pink if you prefer.

Low-Carb Sweeteners. You now know sugar is 100 percent carbohydrates and should be avoided, so what can you use to sweeten things up? You have a couple of low-carb alternatives. The most obvious is artificial sweetener. Brands like Splenda make products that can be used exactly like sugar (swapped measure for measure in cooking and baking). If you're not sure how you feel about artificial sweetener, you can use naturally sweet foods like berries to sweeten foods like yogurt. The good news is that as you get used to eating low-carb, you will crave sugar less and less and a little bit will go a long way.

Low-Carb Thickeners. A nice hearty soup or stew can be so comforting, but most people use flour or cornstarch to thicken them (both high-carb options). When cooking at home, you have some alternatives that will thicken your dish with fewer carbs. One option is to purée the food using an immersion blender. This works especially well with soups—a few pulses of the blender will yield a thicker broth. Another option is to stir in some regular cream or sour cream, which can lend a thicker, creamier consistency to dishes.

10 Tips for Dining Out

You aren't stuck dining at home just because you've gone low-carb. You just need a game plan before heading out to any of your favorite restaurants.

1. **Don't tempt yourself.** Are you the kind of person who can sit in a pizza restaurant, smelling all that delicious dough, and order a salad? Can you go to an Italian restaurant, see everyone around you slurping spaghetti, and abstain? If you're not, don't put yourself in that situation. Tell your friends and family that you're trying to eat fewer carbs and they will most likely be totally fine with going to a different dining destination. Once you're more comfortable with low-carb eating and don't crave bad-for-you fare anymore, you can hit up the pizza parlor without fear.

2. **Head online before leaving the house.** Many chain restaurants and fast-food joints have all their nutritional information listed online. Check out the menu for a few minutes before leaving home, and you'll know what dishes have sneaky carbs in them and which ones are smart choices.

3. **Ask for substitutions.** Just because your roast chicken comes with mashed potatoes doesn't mean you can't ask for spinach or broccoli instead. Even sandwich shops usually have the option of getting the fillings on a bed of lettuce instead of a sub roll. Getting guacamole? Ask if you can have the carrots and celery that come with the chicken wings instead of tortilla chips. Don't be shy. Waiters are used to getting requests from diners and want you to enjoy your meal. You never know what they can adjust for you if you don't ask.

4. **Police your portions.** If 1 cup of soup you make yourself has 10 grams of carbohydrates, you aren't doing too much damage. But go to a restaurant and eat the 3-cup bowl and all of a sudden you're putting a big dent in your daily allowance. Portion sizes at restaurants are totally out of balance with how much you actually should be eating. Get around it by ordering an appetizer as your main course or by eating only half your entrée and saving the rest for another meal.

5. **Get sauces on the side.** Salad dressing, barbecue sauce, and almost every other sweet condiment might add a ton of flavor, but they're also packed with sugar and carbs. You don't have to eat a bland chicken breast, but get the sauce on the side, dip your fork in it, and then pierce your food. You'll get the flavor you like but limit the carbs.

6. **Banish the breadbasket.** Dinners rolls, biscuits, and focaccia are amazing and come free at almost every restaurant in America. But does that mean you should begin your meal with them? Absolutely not. Instead of staring at all that bread while starving and waiting for your food to arrive, just ask your waiter not to bring it. Problem solved.

7. **Order water only.** When you eat out at a restaurant, you're already taking a gamble by not knowing exactly what ingredients are going into your food. Don't add insult to injury by drinking sugary beverages all meal long. Sodas, sweet iced teas, and cocktails may be listed on the menu, but you don't have to order them.

8. **Have some go-to dishes.** Menus can be confusing. Keep in mind a few dishes that you know are pretty safe—like surf 'n' turf with steak and grilled shrimp, turkey burgers without the bun, and fried eggs with bacon. Then, when all else fails, you can order one of those dishes and feel confident in your decision.

9. **Avoid anything fried.** While the frying itself doesn't boost the carb count, the breading bath the food goes through before hitting the hot oil sure does. Mozzarella cheese may be low-carb, but mozzarella sticks aren't. Same goes for chicken fingers, onion rings, and chicken-fried steak.

10. **Don't be fooled by the salads.** Many people think that if they order a salad, they will be dining practically carb-free. But while some salads are definitely nutrition all-stars, you can't just assume. Watch out for croutons, starchy vegetables, sweet dressings, and other high-carb ingredients. A simple salad can have more than 100 grams of carbs if you don't pay attention to ingredients. This is when it's time to customize and ask the waiter to do some simple swaps.

CHAPTER FIVE

14-Day Meal Plan

Congratulations! You're now armed with all the information, tips, tricks, and numbers needed to begin your very own low-carb diet. What follows is a 14-day meal plan showing you just how delicious and easy low-carb cooking can be. Each day includes a breakfast, midmorning snack, lunch, afternoon snack, dinner, and dessert. As you'll see, this is not a diet where you're going to be hungry and cranky all the time.

Beginning a diet is often the hardest part, so think of this meal plan as your personal coach over the next two weeks. At the end of this period, you'll be so used to low-carb eating and so comfortable cooking this way, you'll be good to go off and create your own low-carb meal plan every day. You should, however, continue to keep a food log of what you eat and how many carbs are in your meals, just so you don't start to veer off course or return to your old ways.

A few other thoughts: The dishes are, for the most part, relatively simple to prepare (the recipes marked with an asterisk are from this cookbook). They are completely customizable and swappable—this is just to give you an idea of how your days should look moving forward so you can get started. A total carb count (gross carbs) is given for one serving of each dish. A daily total is also provided—each menu delivers fewer than 100 grams of carbs per day.

Day 1   *Breakfast*: Scrambled Eggs with Lox and Cream Cheese* (3.5 grams; page 40)
Midmorning snack: ¼ cup almonds and ½ orange (14.5 grams)
Lunch: Creamy Tomato Soup* (13 grams; page 74)
Afternoon snack: ½ cup low-fat cottage cheese and 1 cup fresh strawberries (15 grams)
Dinner: 3-ounce baked chicken breast with 1½ cups Brussels sprouts roasted in 1 tablespoon olive oil (12 grams)
Dessert: ½ cup chocolate ice cream (15 grams)
TOTAL CARBS: 73 grams

Day 2 *Breakfast*: 2 scrambled eggs and 1 chicken sausage (12 grams)
Midmorning snack: 1 cup low-fat cottage cheese with ½ cup fresh cantaloupe (15.5 grams)
Lunch: Spicy Shrimp and Black Bean Salad* (19 grams; page 105)
Afternoon snack: 2 cups baked kale chips made with 1 tablespoon olive oil (13.5 grams)
Dinner: Stir-Fry with Greens and Walnuts* (11 grams; page 123)
Dessert: 1 packet sugar-free hot cocoa made with hot water (10 grams)
TOTAL CARBS: 81 grams

Day 3 *Breakfast*: 1 cup plain Greek yogurt with 1 tablespoon almonds and ½ cup raspberries (18 grams)
Midmorning snack: 2 hard-boiled eggs with salt and pepper (1 gram)
Lunch: Butternut Squash Bisque* (12 grams; page 76)
Afternoon snack: 4 slices deli turkey wrapped around ½ cucumber cut into spears (6 grams)
Dinner: Fajita Salad* (13 grams; page 107)
Dessert: Fudge Popsicle (12 grams)
TOTAL CARBS: 62 grams

Day 4 *Breakfast*: Strawberry and Tofu Smoothie* (11 grams; page 35)
Midmorning snack: ½ cup plain Greek yogurt with ¼ cup sliced grapes (11.5 grams)
Lunch: 2 cups arugula salad with 2 ounces prosciutto, 1 large cantaloupe wedge, and lemon vinaigrette made with 1 tablespoon olive oil and 1 tablespoon lemon juice (13.5 grams)
Afternoon snack: ½ fresh pear and ¼ cup sunflower seeds (18.5 grams)
Dinner: Turkey Meatloaf* (13 grams; page 155)
Dessert: 1 cup ricotta cheese with 1 tablespoon sugar-free vanilla syrup and 1 teaspoon ground cinnamon (9.5 grams)
TOTAL CARBS: 77 grams

Day 5 *Breakfast*: 2-egg omelet with ½ cup broccoli, ½ cup green bell pepper, and ¼ cup Cheddar cheese (5 grams)
Midmorning snack: ½ fresh pear and 2 slices Cheddar cheese (11.5 grams)
Lunch: Miso and Clam Soup* (5 grams; page 81)
Afternoon snack: 2 stalks celery with 2 tablespoons hummus (8.5 grams)
Dinner: 4 ounces pan-seared flank steak with 2 cups roasted cauliflower (10.5 grams)
Dessert: Almond Cheesecake Bars* (15 grams; page 186)
TOTAL CARBS: 55.5 grams

Day 6   *Breakfast*: 1 cup plain Greek yogurt with ½ cup fresh blueberries (19.5 grams)
Midmorning snack: 1 hard-boiled egg with ½ apple (13 grams)
Lunch: Thai Soup with Coconut and Tofu* (15 grams; page 80)
Afternoon snack: 2 large pieces beef jerky (4.5 grams)
Dinner: Cheeseburger-Stuffed Peppers* (9.5 grams; page 163)
Dessert: 1 ounce dark chocolate (17 grams)
TOTAL CARBS: 78.5 grams

Day 7   *Breakfast*: Cottage Cheese Pancakes* (11 grams; page 39)
Midmorning snack: 2 stalks celery with 2 tablespoons peanut butter (11 grams)
Lunch: 1 cup canned Italian wedding soup with meatballs (20 grams)
Afternoon snack: 8 slices pepperoni and 2 ounces Cheddar cheese (1 gram)
Dinner: Cioppino* (15 grams; page 84)
Dessert: ½ banana with 1 tablespoon chocolate-hazelnut spread (24.5 grams)
TOTAL CARBS: 82.5 grams

Day 8   *Breakfast*: ½ avocado, ½ tomato, sliced, with 2 scrambled eggs and ¼ cup shredded Cheddar cheese (11.5 grams)
Midmorning snack: 1 string cheese and ½ apple (13 grams)
Lunch: 2 cups mixed greens with ¼ cup feta, 3 ounces grilled chicken breast, and 2 tablespoons sliced olives (5.5 grams)
Afternoon snack: Hot and Smoky Nuts* (6.5 grams; page 54)
Dinner: 4-ounce cheeseburger with no bun and 1 cup sautéed spinach (7 grams)
Dessert: Spiced Pears* (20 grams; page 175)
TOTAL CARBS: 63.5 grams

Day 9   *Breakfast*: 1 cup low-fat cottage cheese with 1 peach, sliced (19 grams)
Midmorning snack: ½ banana and 1 string cheese (13.5 grams)
Lunch: Fish Tacos with Mango Salsa* (15 grams; page 143)
Afternoon snack: 4 tomato slices topped with 4 slices whole milk mozzarella and 2 tablespoons chopped fresh basil (6.5 grams)
Dinner: Classic Chili* (5 grams; page 88)
Dessert: Sugar-free chocolate pudding cup (13 grams per 3.25-ounce cup)
TOTAL CARBS: 72 grams

14-Day Meal Plan

Day 10 *Breakfast*: Hot Breakfast Cereal with Flaxseed* (17 grams; page 37)
Midmorning snack: 3 tablespoons trail mix with peanuts, dark
chocolate chips, raisins, almonds, and cashews (12 grams)
Lunch: Chef's salad made with 2 cups lettuce, 3 slices deli turkey,
3 slices deli ham, 2 slices Swiss cheese, and 2 slices Cheddar
cheese (7 grams)
Afternoon snack: Tuna salad made with ½ can tuna, 1 tablespoon
light mayonnaise, and ¼ cup diced celery, served with 1 cup cucumber
slices (6 grams)
Dinner: Pizza with Cauliflower Crust* (14 grams; page 126)
Dessert: ½ cup chocolate ice cream (15 grams)
TOTAL CARBS: 71 grams

Day 11 *Breakfast*: 2 fried eggs and 2 slices of bacon (1 gram)
Midmorning snack: 1 cup plain Greek yogurt with ½ cup sliced
strawberries (14.5 grams)
Lunch: Caesar Salad with Mushrooms* (10 grams; page 98)
Afternoon snack: 2 tablespoons hummus with 1 cup carrot strips and
12 baby tomatoes (21.5 grams)
Dinner: Salmon with Miso and Ginger* (6 grams; page 146)
Dessert: 1 ounce dark chocolate (17 grams)
TOTAL CARBS: 70 grams

Day 12 *Breakfast*: Open-Face Omelet with Goat Cheese, Spinach, and
Sun-Dried Tomatoes* (3 grams; page 42)
Midmorning snack: Large cappuccino with whole milk (12 grams)
Lunch: Open-faced sandwich with 1 slice whole-wheat bread,
2 tablespoons peanut butter, and 1 tablespoon sugar-free jelly served
with 1 cup snap peas (27.5 grams)
Afternoon snack: 4 slices deli ham wrapped around ½ cup fresh
pineapple chunks (10.5 grams)
Dinner: Braised Pork Chops with Fennel* (13.5 grams; page 158)
Dessert: 13 chocolate-covered almonds (18 grams)
TOTAL CARBS: 84.5 grams

Day 13 *Breakfast*: 2 ounces smoked salmon and 2 poached eggs (1 gram)
Midmorning snack: 10 baby carrots dipped in 2 tablespoons ranch
dressing (9.5 grams)
Lunch: Multigrain tortilla wrap with 3 ounces grilled chicken, ¼ cup
alfalfa sprouts, and ¼ avocado, sliced (21.5 grams)

Afternoon snack: Spicy Popcorn* (6.5 grams; page 53)
Dinner: 2 cups roasted spaghetti squash with ½ cup spaghetti sauce (31 grams)
Dessert: Cherry Sorbet* (11 grams; page 172)
TOTAL CARBS: 80.5 grams

Day 14   *Breakfast*: Frittata with Fresh Herbs* (2 grams; page 41)
Midmorning snack: ½ apple with 2 tablespoons almond butter (19.5 grams)
Lunch: Summer Salad with Squash, Beets, and Mushrooms* (8 grams; page 99)
Afternoon snack: ½ cup mixed nuts (17.5 grams)
Dinner: 3 ounces grilled salmon with 2 cups broccoli roasted with 1 tablespoon olive oil (9 grams)
Dessert: Sugar-free strawberry gelatin cup (0 grams)
TOTAL CARBS: 56 grams

Breakfast

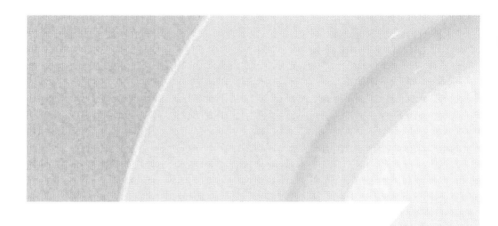

Breakfast

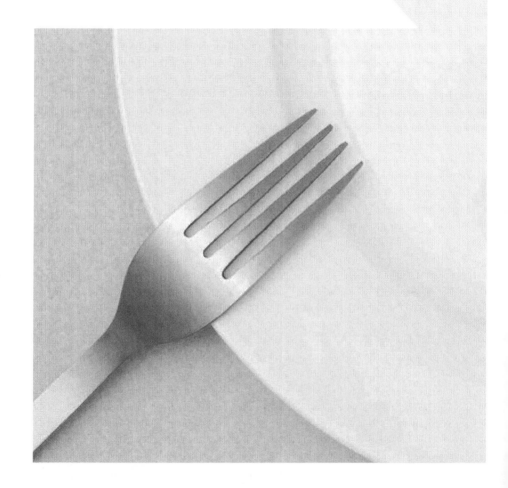

Strawberry and Tofu Smoothie

SERVES 4

On busy mornings, a smoothie can be a quick breakfast option that's easy to take with you. This recipe calls for frozen berries. If you are using fresh, freeze them first to get the right consistency in the final drink.

1 cup frozen strawberries
1 cup ice cubes
½ cup heavy cream
2 tablespoons sugar
3½ ounces soft or silken tofu
½ teaspoon pure vanilla extract

Combine all ingredients in a blender and purée until smooth. Pour evenly into four glasses and serve immediately.

GROSS CARBS **11 G**
NET CARBS **10 G**

Breakfast

Granola with Coconut and Cherries

MAKES 28 SERVINGS

This recipe makes almost 7 cups of granola, so it might make sense to freeze some (unless you're serving it to a crowd). Store it in an airtight container in the freezer for up to 1 month.

2¾ cups rolled oats
1 cup unsweetened coconut flakes
1 cup unsalted shelled pistachios
⅓ cup unsalted pepitas (pumpkin seeds)
1½ teaspoons salt
½ cup packed light brown sugar
⅓ cup pure maple syrup
⅓ cup olive oil
¾ cup dried cherries

Preheat the oven to 300°F. Line two baking sheets with parchment paper.

In a large bowl, mix together the oats, coconut, pistachios, pepitas, and salt. In a small saucepan over low heat, add the brown sugar, maple syrup, and olive oil, and warm, stirring until the sugar dissolves. Fold the sugar mixture into the oat mixture to evenly coat.

Spread the granola on the prepared baking sheets and bake for 20 to 25 minutes, stirring often, until dry and golden brown. Remove from the oven and toss with the dried cherries. Let cool to room temperature.

GROSS CARBS: **10 G**
NET CARBS: **8 G**

Hot Breakfast Cereal with Flaxseed

SERVES 1

When the weather gets cold, a warm breakfast cereal can be just what you're craving. Skip the packets of oatmeal—those are often packed with sugar and carbs. This version has nutrient-rich flaxseed instead and is packed with 12 grams of fiber.

¼ cup ground flaxseed
½ cup boiling water
¼ teaspoon cinnamon
Pinch of nutmeg
2 tablespoons applesauce
2 tablespoons almond butter
¼ cup unsweetened almond milk

In a small bowl, cover the ground flaxseed with the boiling water. Add the cinnamon and nutmeg and stir well. Add the applesauce and almond butter and mix well. Pour the almond milk over top and enjoy immediately.

GROSS CARBS **17 G**
NET CARBS **5 G**

Blueberry Biscuits

MAKES 12

The flavor of fresh fruit shines through in this easy recipe that has all the taste of classic blueberry muffins. No fresh blueberries at the store? Frozen ones work just as well—use them straight from the freezer without allowing them to thaw.

Cooking spray for baking sheet
1 cup all-purpose flour
½ teaspoon salt
1½ teaspoons baking powder
2 tablespoons butter, cut into small pieces
½ cup milk
½ cup blueberries

Preheat the oven to 350°F. Coat a baking sheet with cooking spray.

In a large bowl, combine the flour, salt, and baking powder. Add the butter and, using a pastry cutter or two knives, cut it into the flour mixture. Stir in the milk, then fold in the blueberries. Drop by heaped tablespoonfuls onto the prepared baking sheet. Bake for 12 to 14 minutes or until lightly browned.

GROSS CARBS: **9.5 G**

NET CARBS: **9 G**

Cottage Cheese Pancakes

While classic pancakes are a breakfast staple, they don't tend to show up in low-carb cookbooks. This version is packed with protein from the cottage cheese and eggs and tastes surprisingly like the real thing. Serve with fresh fruit on top.

1 cup low-fat cottage cheese
⅓ cup all-purpose flour
2 tablespoons vegetable oil
3 eggs, lightly beaten
Cooking spray for pan

In a large bowl, combine the cottage cheese, flour, oil, and eggs. Coat a large skillet or sauté pan with cooking spray and heat over medium heat. Pour ⅓ cup of the batter onto the pan and cook until bubbles appear on the surface, about 2 minutes. Flip the pancake over and cook until browned on the other side, another 1 or 2 minutes.

GROSS CARBS: **11 G**
NET CARBS: **10.5 G**

Scrambled Eggs with Lox and Cream Cheese

SERVES 6

Leave the bagel out of this classic breakfast dish—you'll never miss it with so many other flavors happening. Add chopped fresh chives, capers, thinly sliced red onion, or tomato if you'd like. And make sure the cream cheese is very cold when you fold it in, so chunks appear throughout the final dish.

12 eggs
½ teaspoon salt
½ teaspoon pepper
3 tablespoons butter
8 ounces cold cream cheese, cut into ½-inch cubes
6 ounces cold-smoked salmon (lox), thinly sliced and
        cut into ½-inch-wide strips

In a large bowl, whisk together the eggs, salt, and pepper.

In a large nonstick skillet or sauté pan over medium-high heat, melt the butter. Add the eggs and stir until almost set, about 5 minutes. Fold in the cheese and salmon and stir just until the eggs are set, about 1 minute more. Serve immediately.

GROSS CARBS: **3.5 G**
NET CARBS: **3.5 G**

Low-Carb Cookbook

Frittata with Fresh Herbs

Using fresh herbs like parsley and dill is a healthful way to boost the flavor of a dish without adding fat, calories, or sodium. Instead of the dill, you can substitute basil, chives, or any other herb you like. Make sure to use unsalted butter, or the dish will turn out too salty.

10 eggs
Dash of salt
Dash of pepper
2 tablespoons chopped fresh dill
2 tablespoons chopped fresh flat-leaf parsley
2 tablespoons unsalted butter
8 ounces low-fat sour cream

Preheat the oven to 350°F.

In a large bowl, beat the eggs with the salt, pepper, dill, and parsley.

In a medium ovenproof skillet or sauté pan over medium-low heat, melt the butter until it begins to foam. Swirl the melted butter to coat the bottom and sides of the pan. Add the egg mixture and immediately transfer the pan to oven. Bake for 10 minutes.

Remove from the oven and let rest for 5 minutes. Invert the frittata onto a plate and serve it with sour cream on the side.

GROSS CARBS: **2 G**
NET CARBS: **2 G**

Open-Face Omelet with Goat Cheese, Spinach, and Sun-Dried Tomatoes

SERVES 4

The hardest part about making an omelet can be the flipping and folding of the eggs. This recipe takes that step out and keeps things easier, resulting in an open-faced version full of Italian flavors.

2 tablespoons butter
8 sun-dried tomatoes packed in oil, drained and finely chopped
2 green onions, thinly sliced (white and green parts)
Salt and pepper
2 cups gently packed baby spinach, coarsely chopped
6 eggs
2 ounces goat cheese, crumbled

In a large nonstick ovenproof skillet or sauté pan over medium heat, melt the butter. Stir in the sun-dried tomatoes and green onions and cook, stirring, until the green onions are wilted, 1 or 2 minutes. Season with salt and pepper. Stir in the spinach and cook until it's wilted and the moisture is evaporated, about 4 minutes.

In a medium bowl, beat the eggs. Season with salt and pepper.

Reduce heat to medium-low. Pour in the eggs and cook until they start to set around the edges, 1 or 2 minutes. Using a spatula, push some of the cooked egg from the edge toward the center, letting the unset egg fill in the hole you made. Repeat all the way around the edge.

Scatter the goat cheese on top of the omelet.

Turn the oven to broil and position an oven rack 5 inches below the broiler. Place the pan under the broiler, leaving the oven door ajar, and cook until the top of the omelet is set, about 2 minutes, watching constantly to make sure the omelet doesn't get too brown. Serve immediately.

GROSS CARBS: **3 G**
NET CARBS: **2 G**

Breakfast "Burrito"

SERVES 4

This dish has all the flavors of the classic Southwest recipe, but without the carbohydrate-rich flour tortilla. In its place is a super-thin layer of scrambled eggs. A few slices of avocado or tomato would be a perfect accompaniment.

1 cup canned black beans, drained and rinsed
⅓ cup bottled salsa
4 eggs
2 tablespoons milk
¼ teaspoon pepper
⅛ teaspoon salt
Cooking spray for pan
½ cup shredded Monterey Jack cheese
¼ cup low-fat sour cream

In a small saucepan, mash the beans slightly. Mix in the salsa.

Place the beans over low heat, and cook until thoroughly warm. Remove from the heat and cover to keep warm.

In a medium bowl, beat the eggs, milk, pepper, and salt. Coat a medium nonstick skillet or sauté pan with cooking spray and heat over medium heat. Pour ¼ cup of the egg mixture into the pan. Lift and tilt the pan to spread the egg mixture evenly over the bottom. Return to the heat and cook until lightly browned on bottom, 1½ to 2 minutes.

Without flipping, loosen the edges of the egg tortilla with a spatula and slide it out onto a serving plate. Spread one-fourth of the warm bean mixture over half of the tortilla. Top the beans with the cheese. Fold the plain egg half over the beans-and-cheese half of the egg tortilla. Repeat with the remaining egg mixture, to make three other egg tortillas. Serve with sour cream.

GROSS CARBS: **15 G**
NET CARBS: **12 G**

Eggs, Swiss Chard, and Mushroom Sauté

SERVES 2

Swiss chard is full of vitamin A, vitamin C, and antioxidants. It also comes in many different colors—orange, red, and even a rainbow variety—but they all taste similar. If you can't find Swiss chard, you can substitute spinach.

1 pound Swiss chard
2 tablespoons olive oil
1 medium onion, chopped
6 shiitake mushrooms, cut into ¼-inch-thick slices
Salt and pepper
4 eggs

Cut the chard leaves off the center rib. Cut the ribs into ½-inch pieces and cut the leaves crosswise into 1-inch ribbons.

In a large, nonstick lidded skillet or sauté pan, heat the oil over medium-high heat. Add the onion, chard ribs, and mushrooms. Sauté until the onion is translucent, 4 to 5 minutes. Add the chard leaves and stir. Season with salt and pepper.

Spread the mixture evenly in the pan. Crack the eggs one at a time onto the vegetable mixture. Reduce the heat to low and cover the pan. Cook until the egg whites are cooked through, 3 to 4 minutes. Serve immediately.

GROSS CARBS: **24.5 G**
NET CARBS: **17.5 G**

Baked Eggs in Ham Cups

SERVES 3

This kid-friendly breakfast uses muffin tins to create little ham cups, which then hold the egg mixture. When cooking this dish, if the eggs begin to brown too much in the oven, cover the muffin tin with aluminum foil for the remainder of the baking time.

Cooking spray for muffin tin
6 slices of deli ham
6 eggs
1 tablespoon milk
¼ teaspoon salt
¼ teaspoon pepper
1 green onion, finely chopped
¼ green bell pepper, finely chopped
2 tablespoons chopped olives
½ teaspoon dried marjoram
⅓ cup grated Cheddar cheese

Preheat the oven to 375°F. Coat six standard muffin cups with cooking spray.

Line each muffin cup with 1 slice of the ham.

In a medium bowl, beat the eggs, milk, salt, and pepper. Fold in the green onion, bell pepper, olives, marjoram, and Cheddar.

Spoon ½ cup of the egg mixture into each of the six muffin cups. Bake for 20 to 25 minutes or until the eggs are set. Remove from the oven and run a knife around the sides of the muffin cups to loosen the baked eggs. Serve immediately.

GROSS CARBS: **6.5 G**
NET CARBS: **6 G**

Crust-Free Quiche with Cheese and Bacon

There's no denying that quiche is delicious, but the standard buttery crust is anything but low-carb. This crustless version is so delicious you'll never miss the pastry. The recipe is completely customizable—swap out bacon and put in cooked crumbled sausage if you'd like or leave the meat out completely to make a vegetarian dish.

4 tablespoons unsalted butter, plus more for pie plate
¼ cup all-purpose flour
¾ cup milk
1 cup low-fat cottage cheese
½ teaspoon baking powder
½ teaspoon salt
½ teaspoon Dijon mustard
5 eggs
4 ounces cream cheese, softened
6 ounces Swiss cheese, shredded
3 tablespoons grated Parmesan cheese
3 slices bacon, cooked and crumbled
6 cherry tomatoes, halved

In a medium saucepan over medium heat, melt the butter. Add the flour and cook, stirring until bubbly. Gradually add the milk and cook, stirring constantly until the sauce thickens, 1 to 2 minutes. Remove the sauce from the heat and set aside to cool for 15 to 20 minutes.

Preheat the oven to 350°F. Butter a 10-inch pie plate.

In a medium bowl, combine the cottage cheese, baking powder, salt, and Dijon mustard.

In a large bowl, beat the eggs. Add the cream cheese to the eggs and stir until combined. Stir in the cottage cheese mixture and the butter sauce into the egg mixture. Fold in the Swiss and Parmesan cheeses.

Pour the mixture into the prepared pie plate. Sprinkle with the bacon and tomatoes. Bake until lightly browned on top and a knife inserted into the center comes out clean, about 40 minutes. Let rest for 15 minutes before serving.

GROSS CARBS: **7.5 G**
NET CARBS: **7 G**

Egg-Stuffed Mushrooms

SERVES 2

Portobello mushrooms (basically overgrown cremini mushrooms) are full of hearty flavor and are a great source of fiber. Here they become a vessel for Mediterranean-style scrambled eggs. While the recipe calls for egg substitute, you can swap in two whole eggs instead.

2 portobello mushrooms, stemmed
Cooking spray for coating the mushrooms
⅛ teaspoon garlic salt
⅛ teaspoon pepper
½ teaspoon olive oil
1 small onion, finely chopped
1 cup gently packed baby spinach
½ cup egg substitute
⅛ teaspoon salt
¼ cup crumbled feta cheese
2 tablespoons finely chopped fresh basil

Preheat the oven to 425°F.

Coat the mushrooms with cooking spray. Sprinkle them with the garlic salt and a dash of the pepper. Transfer to a baking sheet and bake for 10 minutes or until tender.

In a large saucepan, heat the olive oil over medium heat. Add the onion and sauté until tender, 3 to 4 minutes. Stir in the spinach and cook, tossing until wilted.

In a small bowl, whisk the egg substitute, salt, and the remaining pepper. Add the egg mixture to the pan and cook until set, stirring occasionally.

Divide the egg mixture among the mushroom caps and sprinkle with the feta and basil. Serve warm.

GROSS CARBS: **10 G**
NET CARBS: **7 G**

Cauliflower Hash Browns

SERVES 4

Cauliflower masquerades as potatoes in this all-American breakfast side. Serve with two fried eggs for a meal that will keep you feeling satisfied until lunchtime.

1 head cauliflower
8 slices bacon, chopped
1 cup chopped onion
2 tablespoons butter, at room temperature, cut into 8 pieces
Salt and pepper

Using a cheese grater placed over a large bowl, grate the cauliflower.

In a large skillet or sauté pan over medium high heat, cook the bacon and onion until they start to brown, about 10 minutes. Add the grated cauliflower. Cook, stirring regularly, until the cauliflower is tender and browned all over. While the cauliflower is cooking, add pieces of the butter every few minutes until the butter is incorporated. Season with salt and pepper. Serve warm.

GROSS CARBS: **11.5 G**

NET CARBS: **7 G**

Turkey and Apple Breakfast Sausage

SERVES 4

This quick sausage is made using ground turkey instead of ground pork, which is higher in fat. Opt for all-white-meat ground turkey for an even leaner option.

½ apple, peeled, cored, and shredded
¼ cup finely chopped almonds or pecans
1½ teaspoons finely chopped fresh sage
¼ teaspoon black pepper
⅛ teaspoon salt
⅛ teaspoon paprika
⅛ teaspoon cayenne pepper
Dash of ground nutmeg
8 ounces ground turkey
Cooking spray for broiler pan

In a large bowl, combine the apple, almonds, sage, pepper, salt, paprika, cayenne pepper, and nutmeg. Add the ground turkey and mix well. Shape into four ½-inch-thick patties.

Place the turkey patties on a broiler pan coated with cooking spray. Turn on the broiler, place an oven rack about 5 inches from the broiler, and broil the patties for 10 minutes or until lightly browned and no longer pink inside (a thermometer should read 165°F), flipping once halfway through the cooking time.

GROSS CARBS: **5 G**
NET CARBS: **3.5 G**

Snacks and Appetizers

Spicy Popcorn

Hot and Smoky Nuts

Hummus

Crab Dip

Curried Deviled Eggs

Artichoke Heart Bites

Shrimp Cocktail

Coconut Shrimp

Smoked Salmon Rolled with Basil and Crème Fraiche

Chicken Skewers with Tomato, Lemon, and Rosemary

Asian Turkey Meatballs

Classic Buffalo Wings with Blue Cheese Dip

Melon, Prosciutto, and Mozzarella Skewers

Bacon-Stuffed Mushrooms

Scotch Eggs

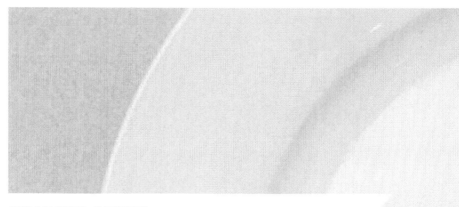

Snacks and Appetizers

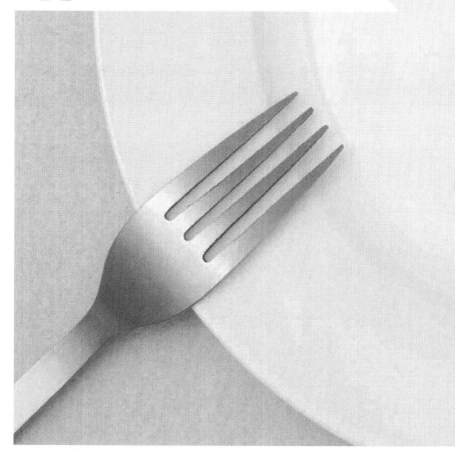

Spicy Popcorn

The next time you stay in to watch movies, make up a batch of this super flavorful popcorn. Instead of plain butter and salt, give the popped corn a sprinkling of chili powder, cumin, cayenne, and cinnamon. Make the popcorn however you'd like, but try not to use any extra butter in the popping process.

½ teaspoon ground cumin
½ teaspoon chili powder
½ teaspoon salt
Dash of cayenne pepper
Dash of ground cinnamon
12 cups freshly popped popcorn
Cooking spray for coating popcorn

In a small bowl, combine the cumin, chili powder, salt, cayenne pepper, and cinnamon.

Spread the popped popcorn in an even layer in a large shallow baking pan. Lightly coat with cooking spray and sprinkle evenly with the spice mixture. Toss to coat well.

GROSS CARBS: **6.5 G**
NET CARBS: **5 G**

53

Snacks and Appetizers

Hot and Smoky Nuts

SERVES 12

Spiced nuts are a tasty source of protein. This version mixes sweet and spicy flavors, making the nuts an irresistible snack. Once cool, the nuts can be stored in an airtight container at room temperature for up to 3 days.

1 tablespoon butter, melted

2 tablespoons Worcestershire sauce

4 teaspoons chili powder

4 teaspoons reduced-sodium soy sauce

1 tablespoon hot pepper sauce

2 garlic cloves, minced

1 tablespoon packed light brown sugar

¼ teaspoon ground cinnamon

3 cups pecan halves

Mesquite or hickory chips for the grill

In a large bowl, combine melted butter, Worcestershire sauce, chili powder, soy sauce, hot pepper sauce, garlic, brown sugar, and cinnamon. Add the nuts and toss to coat. Transfer to a 13-by-9-inch disposable foil baking pan.

To prepare the grill, arrange the mesquite or hickory chips over the charcoal, according to the package instructions.

Grill the nuts in the foil pan over indirect very low heat, stirring occasionally, until the nuts are dry and crisp, about 25 minutes. Watch carefully the last 10 minutes so the nuts don't burn.

GROSS CARBS: **6.5 G**

NET CARBS: **3.5 G**

Hummus

In the past decade, this chickpea dip has gone from specialty-store find to mainstream staple. Tahini is a sesame seed paste that can often be found in the international food section of the supermarket. Make sure to give it a good stir before using, since the paste tends to separate when sitting around.

2 cups canned garbanzo beans (chickpeas), drained and rinsed
⅓ cup tahini
¼ cup lemon juice
1 teaspoon salt
2 garlic cloves, halved
1 tablespoon extra-virgin olive oil
Pinch of paprika
1 teaspoon minced fresh parsley

In a food processor, blend the garbanzo beans, tahini, lemon juice, salt, and garlic until smooth. Transfer to a medium bowl. Drizzle with the olive oil and sprinkle with the paprika and parsley.

55

GROSS CARBS: **16.5 G**
NET CARBS: **13 G**

Snacks and Appetizers

Crab Dip

You don't need to live in Maryland or Alaska to be able to cook up a delicious crab dip. Most grocery stores sell cooked crabmeat in jars in the seafood refrigerated section. Before using, make sure you go through it with your fingers to discard any leftover pieces of shell.

½ cup light mayonnaise
½ cup low-fat sour cream
2 tablespoons minced shallot
½ teaspoon dried dill
1 teaspoon grated lemon zest
1 teaspoon lemon juice
1 teaspoon white wine vinegar
½ teaspoon Worcestershire sauce
1 cup cooked crabmeat
Salt and pepper

In a medium bowl, combine the mayonnaise, sour cream, shallots, dill, lemon zest, lemon juice, white wine vinegar, and Worcestershire sauce. Fold in the crabmeat and season with salt and pepper. Chill for 2 hours or overnight. Serve with veggies and crackers.

GROSS CARBS: **1 G**
NET CARBS: **1 G**

Curried Deviled Eggs

This all-American appetizer is naturally low-carb. It can be made up to 8 hours ahead of time—just cover and refrigerate. The deviled eggs can be garnished with olives if you'd like.

6 hard-boiled eggs, shelled
¼ cup light mayonnaise
1 tablespoon minced green onion (white and green parts)
¾ teaspoon curry powder
Salt and pepper
1 tablespoon minced fresh parsley

Cut the hard-boiled eggs in half lengthwise, and place on a plate.

Scoop the yolks into a medium bowl and mash them with a fork. Add the mayonnaise, minced green onion, and curry powder. Mix well. Season with salt and pepper. Divide the filling among the egg halves and sprinkle with parsley.

GROSS CARBS: **1 G**
NET CARBS: **1 G**

Snacks and Appetizers

Artichoke Heart Bites

The most delicious part of the artichoke is the heart, which isn't all that easy to get to. Skip a step and buy oil-marinated artichoke hearts in a jar, then mix them with herbs, cheese, and eggs, and bake for a delicious, warm hors d'oeuvre.

Cooking spray for muffin tin
1 slice whole-wheat bread, crust removed
¼ teaspoon dried oregano
One 6-ounce jar oil-marinated artichoke hearts, drained,
    rinsed, and chopped
⅓ cup grated Parmesan cheese
2 tablespoons chopped fresh flat-leaf parsley
1 tablespoon olive oil
½ small onion, chopped
1 garlic clove, chopped
½ teaspoon salt
¼ teaspoon red pepper flakes
3 eggs

Preheat the oven to 375°F. Coat a standard six-cup muffin tin with cooking spray.

Toast the bread slice in the toaster until crisp. Cut the toast into bite-size pieces and transfer to a medium bowl. Add the oregano, artichoke hearts, Parmesan, and parsley.

In a small skillet or sauté pan over medium heat, heat the oil. Add the onion, garlic, salt, and red pepper flakes and cook until the onion is soft, about 5 minutes. Stir the onion mixture into the artichoke mixture.

In a small bowl, lightly beat the eggs until foamy. Stir into the artichoke mixture. Spoon ¼ cup of the mixture into each cup of the prepared muffin tin. Bake until lightly puffed, golden, and just set in the center, 17 to 20 minutes.

Let cool on a rack for 5 minutes, then remove from muffin tin. Serve warm.

GROSS CARBS: **8.5 G**
NET CARBS: **7.5 G**

Shrimp Cocktail

SERVES 8

This classic shrimp cocktail is served with a fresh, homemade cocktail sauce that has a nice, spicy kick of horseradish.

2 pounds 12- to 15-count raw shrimp, peeled, deveined, with
    tails left on
1 tablespoon olive oil
½ teaspoon salt
½ teaspoon pepper

Dipping Sauce
½ cup chili sauce
½ cup ketchup
3 tablespoons prepared horseradish
2 teaspoons lemon juice
½ teaspoon Worcestershire sauce
½ teaspoon hot sauce

Preheat the oven to 400°F.

Place the shrimp in a large bowl and add the olive oil, salt, and pepper. Toss to coat, spread on a baking pan, and roast for 8 to 10 minutes or until pink and firm. Set aside to cool.

To make the dipping sauce: Combine the chili sauce, ketchup, horseradish, lemon juice, Worcestershire sauce, and hot sauce in a medium bowl.

Serve the cooled shrimp with dipping sauce.

GROSS CARBS: **13 G**
NET CARBS: **13 G**

Snacks and Appetizers

Coconut Shrimp

This tropical appetizer has begun showing up on local menus and is a scrumptious way to enjoy shrimp. The coconut married with the honey, citrus, and curry powder in the dipping sauce creates a taste sensation.

Cooking spray for coating baking sheet and shrimp

Dipping Sauce
1 teaspoon curry powder
Pinch of red pepper flakes
1 tablespoon honey
2 teaspoons rice vinegar
Zest of 1 orange
Zest and juice of 1 orange

½ cup flaked unsweetened coconut
6 tablespoons panko bread crumbs
3 tablespoons all-purpose flour
2 egg whites
1 pound 21- to 25-count raw shrimp, peeled, deveined, with tails
    left on, butterflied and patted dry
Salt and pepper

Preheat the oven to 450°F. Coat a rimmed baking sheet with cooking spray.

To make the dipping sauce: Toast the curry and red pepper flakes in a dry saucepan over medium heat for about 1 minute. Add the honey, rice vinegar, and orange zest and juice. Bring to a simmer, stirring occasionally, until the sauce is heated through, 1 to 2 minutes. Remove from the heat and set aside.

Combine the coconut, bread crumbs, and flour in a medium bowl or baking dish. Beat the egg whites in a medium bowl until slightly frothy. Sprinkle the shrimp with salt and pepper. Add the shrimp to the egg whites and toss to coat. Lift each shrimp from the egg whites, letting excess drip off, and coat in the coconut-crumb mixture, pressing to adhere.

Place the shrimp on the prepared baking sheet. Lightly coat the shrimp with cooking spray. Bake the shrimp until they are golden on the outside and opaque in the center, 8 to 10 minutes. Serve hot with the dipping sauce.

GROSS CARBS: **14 G**
NET CARBS: **13 G**

Smoked Salmon Rolled with Basil and Crème Fraiche

SERVES 8

Smoked salmon can be found in the refrigerated-seafood section in most grocery stores or specialty-food stores. If you can't find crème fraîche in your supermarket, sour cream is a delicious substitute. This dish can be made 6 hours ahead—just cover and chill.

Twelve ½-inch slices of smoked salmon
¾ cup crème fraîche
¾ cup chopped fresh basil
Pepper
12 large fresh basil leaves

Place 1 salmon slice on the work surface. Spread 2 teaspoons of the crème fraîche over the salmon slice. Sprinkle with 2 teaspoons of the chopped basil. Sprinkle with pepper. Starting at the short end, roll up the salmon slice, enclosing the filling. Spread 1 teaspoon of the crème fraîche over the top of roll, and sprinkle with 1 teaspoon of the chopped basil. Cut the roll crosswise into 5 slices (keeping the sliced roll together). Repeat with the remaining salmon, crème fraîche, and chopped basil, to make 11 more rolls cut in 5 slices each. Arrange the basil leaves on a serving platter, and top each leaf with 1 sliced salmon roll.

GROSS CARBS: **1 G**
NET CARBS: **1 G**

Snacks and Appetizers

Chicken Skewers with Tomato, Lemon, and Rosemary

SERVES 24

This recipe calls for forty-eight bamboo skewers. When cooking food on a wooden skewer, make sure to soak them in water for at least 30 minutes before assembling. Otherwise you risk the skewers catching on fire.

8 skinless boneless chicken breast halves
1 pint grape tomatoes
1 cup olive oil
1 cup fresh lemon juice
6 bay leaves, broken into small pieces
3 tablespoons chopped fresh rosemary
4 garlic cloves, minced
2 teaspoons hot pepper sauce
Salt and pepper
1 cup light mayonnaise

Cut each chicken breast lengthwise into six thin strips. Thread each strip onto one bamboo skewer, leaving ½ inch of skewer exposed. Press 1 grape tomato onto the end of a skewer. Divide the skewers between two 15-by-10-by-2-inch glass baking dishes, stacking them if necessary.

In a large bowl, whisk together the olive oil, lemon juice, bay leaves, rosemary, garlic, and hot pepper sauce. Pour the marinade over the chicken. Marinate the chicken for 1 hour at room temperature, turning the skewers often.

Preheat the oven to 425°F. Remove the skewers from the marinade and arrange them on two rimmed baking sheets, reserving the marinade. Bake the chicken until cooked through, about 8 minutes.

In a medium saucepan, boil the reserved marinade for 1 minute. Let cool for 15 minutes, strain, and pour ½ cup of the marinade into a medium bowl. Whisk in the mayonnaise and season with salt and pepper. Spoon the remaining marinade over the cooked chicken skewers to moisten and serve them with the mayonnaise sauce.

GROSS CARBS: **3 G**
NET CARBS: **2.5 G**

Asian Turkey Meatballs

Meatballs aren't just for topping spaghetti. This Asian variety has the flavors of ginger, soy sauce, and sesame oil, and they make a very satisfying appetizer. Serve with toothpicks nearby.

1¼ pounds 93% lean ground turkey
¼ cup panko bread crumbs
¼ cup chopped fresh cilantro
1 egg, lightly beaten
3 green onions, chopped (white and light green parts)
1 garlic clove, minced
1 tablespoon minced peeled ginger
1 tablespoon low-sodium soy sauce
2 teaspoons sesame oil
½ teaspoon salt

Lime Sesame Dipping Sauce
¼ cup low-sodium soy sauce
2 teaspoons sesame oil
2 tablespoons fresh lime juice
2 tablespoons water
1 tablespoon diced green onion (white and light green parts)

Preheat the oven to 500°F.

In a large bowl, use your hands to mix the ground turkey, bread crumbs, cilantro, egg, green onions, garlic, ginger, soy sauce, sesame oil, and salt. Take ¼ cup of the mixture, shape it into a ball, and place on a baking dish. Repeat, making meatballs with the remaining mixture. Bake the meatballs for 15 minutes, or until cooked through.

To make the lime sesame dipping sauce: Mix together the soy sauce, sesame oil, lime juice, water, and green onion.

Drizzle the meatballs with 1 tablespoon of the sauce. Serve with the remaining sauce on the side.

GROSS CARBS: **8 G**
NET CARBS: **7.5 G**

Classic Buffalo Wings with Blue Cheese Dip

MAKES 12

This bar snack is traditionally served with celery and carrot sticks to help offset the spiciness of the chicken glaze. The blue cheese dip can be refrigerated for up to 1 week if you don't use it all with the wings. Use it as a dressing for iceberg lettuce.

2 pounds chicken wings (about 12 wings)
3 tablespoons butter, melted
¼ cup hot pepper sauce
1 tablespoon paprika
½ teaspoon salt
½ teaspoon cayenne pepper
¼ teaspoon black pepper

Blue Cheese Dip

½ cup low-fat sour cream
½ cup crumbled blue cheese
½ cup light mayonnaise
1 tablespoon white wine vinegar
1 garlic clove, minced

For each chicken wing, cut off the wing tip and cut the wing in half at the joint. Put the chicken wing pieces in a large ziplock bag.

In a small bowl, stir together the melted butter, hot pepper sauce, paprika, salt, cayenne pepper, and black pepper. Reserve 2 tablespoons of the marinade for later use. Pour the rest of the marinade over the chicken in the plastic bag. Seal the bag and let the chicken marinate at room temperature for 30 minutes. Drain the marinade and discard the bag.

Preheat the broiler. Place an oven rack 4 to 5 inches away from the heat.

Place the wing pieces on the rack of a broiler pan, and broil for 10 minutes on each side, or until the chicken is tender and cooked through.

Meanwhile, to make the blue cheese dip: Combine the sour cream, blue cheese, mayonnaise, white wine vinegar, and garlic in a food processor. Blend until smooth.

Remove the wings from the oven and baste with the 2 tablespoons reserved marinade. Serve the warm wings with the blue cheese dip.

GROSS CARBS: **2 G**

NET CARBS: **1.5 G**

Snacks and Appetizers

Melon, Prosciutto, and Mozzarella Skewers

SERVES 6

Sweet cantaloupe, salty prosciutto, and creamy mozzarella become a force to be reckoned with in this easy, skewered appetizer. The recipe can be prepared 2 hours in advance—just cover and refrigerate. Bring back to room temperature for 15 minutes before serving.

½ cup olive oil
⅓ cup fresh basil leaves
1 shallot, quartered
1 cantaloupe, halved crosswise, seeded, cut into six wedges, and peeled
6 small fresh water-packed mozzarella balls or one 8-ounce ball, drained
6 thin slices prosciutto, cut in half lengthwise
Cracked black pepper

In a food processor on the purée setting, pulse the olive oil, basil, and shallot until the basil and shallot are finely chopped.

Cut each cantaloupe wedge in half crosswise. If using an 8-ounce mozzarella ball, cut it into six cubes. On an 8-inch wooden skewer, place 1 piece cantaloupe, 1 piece prosciutto, 1 piece mozzarella, 1 piece prosciutto, and 1 piece melon. Repeat with five other skewers.

Arrange the skewers on a platter, drizzle with the basil oil, and sprinkle with cracked black pepper.

GROSS CARBS: **10.5 G**
NET CARBS: **10 G**

Bacon-Stuffed Mushrooms

SERVES 12

A big platter of stuffed mushrooms makes any appetizer table look as if it's overflowing with deliciousness. This dish is perfect when you're throwing a party because you can prepare the mushrooms the day before and then bake them just before serving.

8 ounces sliced bacon
Olive oil (if needed)
1 cup chopped onion
One 10-ounce package chopped frozen spinach, thawed,
    squeezed dry
4 ounces feta cheese, crumbled
4 ounces cream cheese, at room temperature
¼ teaspoon red pepper flakes
Salt and pepper
48 button mushrooms (about 2¾ pounds), stemmed

Preheat the oven to 375°F. Line two baking sheets with foil.

In a large heavy skillet or sauté pan over medium heat, cook the bacon until crisp, about 8 minutes. Using a slotted spoon, transfer the bacon to paper towels to drain, and then coarsely crumble. Discard all the bacon fat in the pan but ¼ cup plus 2 teaspoons. Add olive oil, if necessary, to equal that amount.

Heat 2 teaspoons of the reserved bacon fat in a medium heavy skillet or sauté pan over medium heat. Add the onion and sauté until tender, about 5 minutes. Transfer the onion to a medium bowl and let cool. Add the bacon, spinach, feta, cream cheese, and red pepper flakes to the bowl with the onion. Season with salt and pepper.

In a large bowl, toss the mushrooms with the reserved ¼ cup bacon fat. Season with salt and pepper. Place the mushrooms cap-side down in a single layer on the prepared baking sheets. Bake until the centers fill with liquid, about 25 minutes. Turn the mushrooms cap-side up and bake until browned and the liquid evaporates, about 20 more minutes. Turn the mushrooms cap-side down again and spoon 1 heaped teaspoon of filling into each cavity. Bake until heated through, about 10 minutes.

GROSS CARBS: **4 G**
NET CARBS: **2.5 G**

Snacks and Appetizers

Scotch Eggs

A Scotch egg is a hard-boiled egg that's been wrapped in sausage, breaded, and deep-fried. This recipe skips the breading and deep-frying and instead bakes the eggs in the oven. Serve with mustard to cut through the richness of the sausage.

1 pound ground pork sausage
½ cup pork rinds, crushed to a powder
½ cup shredded Cheddar cheese
1 teaspoon garlic powder
¼ cup chopped jalapeño, seeded and deribbed
6 hard-boiled eggs, peeled and patted dry

Preheat the oven to 350°F. Line a baking sheet with parchment paper.

In a large bowl, use your hands to combine the sausage, pork rinds, Cheddar, garlic powder, and jalapeño. Divide the mixture into sixths and mold each section around one of the eggs. Place the eggs on the prepared baking sheet and bake for 30 minutes or until brown and crispy on the outside.

GROSS CARBS: **1.5 G**
NET CARBS: **1.5 G**

CHAPTER EIGHT

Soups and Stews

Gazpacho	Miso and Clam Soup
Italian Vegetable Soup	Tom Yum Soup with Shrimp
French Onion Soup	Italian Egg Drop Soup
Creamy Tomato Soup	Cioppino
Peanut Soup with Curry and Tomatoes	Chicken and Wild Rice Soup
	Chicken Tortilla Soup
Butternut Squash Bisque	Slow Cooker Beef and Vegetable Soup with Beer
Broccoli Cheddar Soup	
Cream of Broccoli and Potato Soup	Classic Chili
	Italian Sausage Soup
Brie and Wild Mushroom Soup	Jambalaya
Thai Soup with Coconut and Tofu	

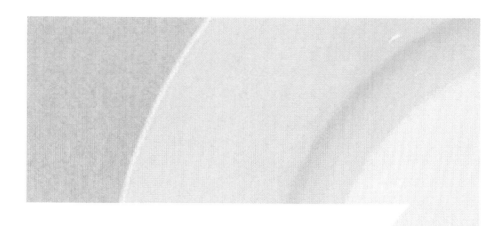

Soups and Stews

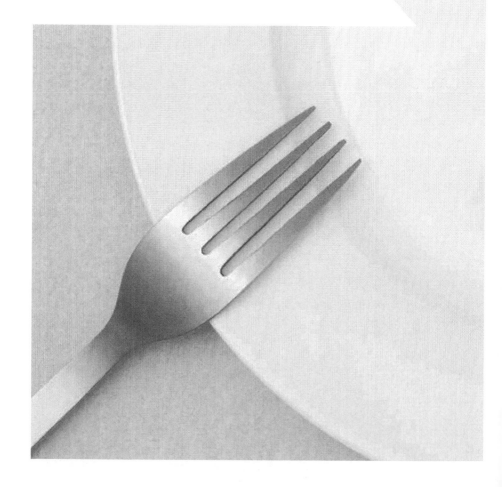

Gazpacho

Gazpacho is a chilled vegetable soup that traditionally has a tomato base. Since you aren't cooking it, the quality of your ingredients is particularly important. Make sure to use only the ripest tomatoes you can find.

2 cups peeled and diced seedless cucumber
2 cups diced red bell pepper
2 cups diced ripe tomato
½ cup diced red onion
2 cups tomato juice
½ cup red wine vinegar
⅓ cup extra-virgin olive oil
2 dashes of Tabasco sauce
Salt and pepper

In a large bowl, combine the cucumber, bell pepper, tomato, and onion. Mix in the tomato juice, vinegar, olive oil, and Tabasco, and season with salt and pepper.

Transfer half the mixture to a blender or food processor and purée (it doesn't have to be perfectly smooth). Return the puréed mixture to the bowl and stir to combine. Refrigerate for 6 hours before serving.

GROSS CARBS: **8 G**
NET CARBS: **6 G**

71

Soups and Stews

Italian Vegetable Soup

To save time, this soup calls for frozen mixed vegetables. Frozen produce is almost always as nutritious as fresh because it is frozen right after picking. There's no need to thaw—keep the vegetables in the freezer until adding them to the soup.

4 cups low-sodium chicken broth
3 cups tomato juice
2 garlic cloves, minced
1 teaspoon dried oregano
¼ teaspoon pepper
16 ounces frozen mixed vegetables (broccoli, cauliflower, and carrots)
One 15-ounce can kidney beans, rinsed and drained

In a soup pot over medium-high heat, combine the chicken broth, tomato juice, garlic, oregano, pepper, and vegetables. Bring to a boil, then reduce heat to low. Cover and cook until the vegetables are tender, about 10 minutes. Add the beans and cook until the mixture is hot and bubbling, 3 to 5 minutes.

GROSS CARBS: **17 G**
NET CARBS: **11 G**

Low-Carb Cookbook

French Onion Soup

SERVES 4

While the classic version of this soup has a crusty slice of bread on top covered in cheese, this recipe skips the bread. You'll never notice it with all the gooey cheese melted over the bowl. If you don't have ramekins, make sure the bowls you use are ovenproof.

2 tablespoons olive oil
3 sweet onions, cut in half and thinly sliced
Two 14.5-ounce cans low-sodium chicken broth
Two 14.5-ounce cans low-sodium beef broth
Dash of sherry
Salt and pepper
4 tablespoons grated Parmesan cheese
8 thin slices provolone cheese
8 thin slices Swiss cheese

In a soup pot over medium-high heat, heat the olive oil and add the onions. Sauté the onions until they are limp and golden brown, about 20 minutes. Add the chicken broth and beef broth and bring to a boil. Add the sherry. Season with salt and pepper.

Preheat the broiler. Place four soup ramekins on a baking sheet.

Ladle the onion broth mixture evenly among the four ramekins. Add 1 tablespoon Parmesan to each bowl of soup and stir gently. Place 2 slices provolone and 2 slices Swiss over each bowl. Keeping the soup bowls on the baking pan, transport them to the oven. Broil until the cheese is golden brown and bubbly, 5 to 10 minutes.

GROSS CARBS: **12.5 G**
NET CARBS: **11 G**

Soups and Stews

Creamy Tomato Soup

SERVES 6

It doesn't get much easier than this soup, which combines cream, basil, and fresh tomatoes. If you don't want to wash a food processor, you can use an immersion blender—just make sure to purée only half the mixture.

One 29-ounce can tomato sauce
4 large tomatoes, peeled and seeded
14 fresh basil leaves
4 tablespoons butter, cubed
1 cup whipping cream
¼ teaspoon salt
¼ teaspoon pepper

In a food processor, combine 1 cup of the tomato sauce, the tomatoes, and basil. Process until puréed. Transfer to a large saucepan and add the butter and remaining tomato sauce.

Over medium-high heat, bring to a boil, reduce the heat to medium-low, and simmer, uncovered, for 15 minutes. Stir in the cream, salt, and pepper and heat through.

GROSS CARBS: **13 G**
NET CARBS: **10 G**

Peanut Soup with Curry and Tomatoes

SERVES 6

If you've never had it before, a soup made with peanut butter can sound strange. But when flavored with curry and cayenne, it turns into something delicious you'd never expect from the sandwich staple.

1 tablespoon olive oil
1 onion, finely chopped
1 green bell pepper, finely chopped
1 celery stalk, finely chopped
1 garlic clove, minced
½ teaspoon curry powder
½ teaspoon paprika
⅛ teaspoon cayenne pepper
1 teaspoon salt, plus more as needed
One 15-ounce can crushed tomatoes
4 cups low-sodium chicken broth
1 teaspoon packed light brown sugar
1 cup water
⅓ cup smooth peanut butter
Pepper

Heat the olive oil in a soup pot over medium-high heat. Add the onion, bell pepper, and celery. Cook, stirring regularly, until the vegetables are softened, about 5 minutes. Add the garlic, curry powder, paprika, cayenne, and salt. Cook, stirring, for 2 minutes more.

Add the tomatoes, chicken broth, brown sugar, and water to the pot. Whisk in the peanut butter until incorporated. Bring to a boil, then reduce the heat to medium-low and simmer gently, stirring occasionally, until the soup thickens slightly, about 30 minutes. Purée with an immersion blender, and season with salt and pepper.

GROSS CARBS: **14 G**
NET CARBS: **11 G**

Butternut Squash Bisque

In the fall and winter, a lack of fresh produce can make it tough to create healthful, vegetable-based meals. That's where butternut squash saves the day. This soup is packed with flavor (thanks in part to the chipotle chiles) and will warm you up on the chilliest of days.

Cooking spray for baking sheet

1½ pounds butternut squash

1 teaspoon canola oil

2 celery stalks, chopped

1 onion, diced

1 carrot, chopped

1 teaspoon ground cumin

¼ teaspoon ground chipotle chile powder

⅛ teaspoon ground cloves

6 cups low-sodium vegetable broth

1 teaspoon salt

¼ teaspoon pepper

½ cup nonfat plain yogurt

2 tablespoons chopped fresh chives

Preheat the oven to 350°F. Coat a rimmed baking sheet lightly with cooking spray.

Cut the squash in half and remove the seeds. Place the halves on the prepared baking sheet, cut-side down. Bake until tender when pierced with a knife, 45 minutes to 1 hour. Let cool and scoop out the flesh.

In a soup pot over medium heat, heat the oil. Add the celery, onion, and carrot. Cover, reduce heat to medium-low, and cook, stirring frequently, until soft, 8 to 10 minutes. Stir in the squash, cumin, ground chipotle, and cloves. Add the broth and simmer, covered, until the vegetables are very tender, 20 to 25 minutes.

Purée the soup with an immersion blender or regular blender until smooth. Add the salt and pepper. Serve garnished with a dollop of yogurt and a sprinkle of chives.

GROSS CARBS: **12 G**

NET CARBS: **9 G**

Broccoli Cheddar Soup

SERVES 8

Even the pickiest of broccoli haters will love this soup, which masks the nutrient-packed vegetable with Cheddar and Parmesan cheeses. Don't be afraid to use the broccoli stems—just peel them first and cut them into smaller pieces.

2 tablespoons unsalted butter
2 pounds broccoli, chopped into 1-inch pieces
1 onion, chopped
2 garlic cloves, minced
1½ teaspoons dry mustard powder
Pinch of cayenne pepper
1 teaspoon salt, plus more as needed
3 cups water
¼ teaspoon baking soda
2 cups chicken broth
2 ounces baby spinach
3 ounces sharp Cheddar cheese, grated
1½ ounces Parmesan cheese, grated
Pepper

In a soup pot over medium-high heat, melt the butter. Add the broccoli, onion, garlic, mustard powder, cayenne, and salt. Cook, stirring frequently, until the vegetables are slightly softened and the mixture is fragrant, about 6 minutes. Add 1 cup of the water and the baking soda and bring to a simmer. Reduce the heat and cook until the broccoli is very soft, about 20 minutes.

Add the broth and the remaining 2 cups water and increase the heat to medium-high. Bring to a simmer, then stir in the spinach and cook until wilted, about 1 minute. Stir in the Cheddar and Parmesan, and blend the soup with an immersion blender. Season with salt and pepper.

GROSS CARBS: **6.5 G**
NET CARBS: **4 G**

Cream of Broccoli and Potato Soup

SERVES 13

Cream of potato soup is delicious, but all that starch can firmly place it on the "avoid" list for low-carbers. Swap out some of the potato for broccoli and you make a huge difference. This recipe serves 13 smaller portions, so use it as an appetizer instead of a main course.

6 cups chicken broth
½ teaspoon pepper
2 garlic cloves, minced
2 heads fresh broccoli, chopped (about 8 cups)
3 potatoes, cut into ¼-inch-thick slices (about 4½ cups)
1 onion, sliced (about 1 cup)
1¾ cups milk
¼ cup grated Parmesan cheese

In a soup pot over high heat, combine the broth, pepper, garlic, broccoli, potatoes, and onion. Bring to a boil, reduce heat to low, cover, and cook for 15 minutes or until vegetables are tender.

Remove the pot from the heat. Using an immersion blender, purée until smooth. Stir in the milk and Parmesan. Cook over medium heat until heated through.

GROSS CARBS: **18 G**

NET CARBS: **14 G**

Brie and Wild Mushroom Soup

SERVES 16

This recipe is definitely more of a first-course soup since it's so rich. A serving should be only about 1/2 cup. Cream sherry is sweeter than regular sherry—if you can't find it, just use regular sherry.

2 cups cream sherry
4 tablespoons butter, cubed
1 pound assorted fresh mushrooms (shiitake, cremini, and oyster)
8 shallots, minced
⅓ cup minced fresh parsley
1 tablespoon lemon juice
⅓ cup all-purpose flour
4 cups beef broth
8 ounces Brie cheese, rind removed, cubed
1 cup heavy cream
1 teaspoon salt
½ teaspoon white pepper

In a small saucepan over medium-high heat, bring the sherry to a boil and cook until reduced by half. Set aside.

In a soup pot, over moderate heat, melt the butter. Add the mushrooms and shallots, and sauté until tender. Add the parsley and lemon juice and stir in. Stir in the flour until well blended. Gradually add the broth and the reduced sherry.

Bring to a boil over medium-high heat. Reduce the heat to medium-low and simmer, uncovered, for 8 to 10 minutes or until thickened. Stir in the Brie and cook, stirring, until melted. Add the cream, salt, and white pepper and heat through, being careful not to boil.

GROSS CARBS: **8 G**
NET CARBS: **7 G**

Thai Soup with Coconut and Tofu

SERVES 6

Thai recipes often include Thai basil. It has a spicier, more peppermint flavor than regular basil and can have a purple or reddish stem. You can find it in specialty grocery stores or you can grow your own.

1 tablespoon vegetable oil
1 stalk lemongrass, white part only, sliced in half lengthwise, cut
    into 6-inch lengths, and smashed with the side of a knife
One 3-inch piece fresh peeled ginger, cut into ½-inch-thick slices
1 jalapeño, halved lengthwise and seeded
4 cups low-sodium chicken broth
One 14-ounce can unsweetened coconut milk
1 tablespoon packed light brown sugar
7 ounces firm tofu, diced
1½ cups frozen peas
6 ounces snow peas, trimmed and strings removed
¼ cup thinly sliced Thai basil leaves
¼ cup fresh lime juice
3 tablespoons fish sauce

In a soup pot over medium-high heat, heat the oil until shimmery. Add the lemongrass, ginger, and jalapeño and cook until fragrant, about 1 minute. Carefully add the broth, coconut milk, and brown sugar and bring to a boil.

Reduce the heat to low and add the tofu, peas, and snow peas. Cook until the snow peas are crisp-tender, about 4 minutes.

Remove from the heat and stir in the basil, lime juice, and fish sauce.

GROSS CARBS: **15 G**
NET CARBS: **12 G**

Low-Carb Cookbook

Miso and Clam Soup

SERVES 4

Dashi granules aren't necessary, but if you can find them, they add a wonderful flavor to this soup. They are made from kelp and dried fish and are sold in specialty stores. Keep in mind that you won't need to add much salt to this soup because miso is naturally salty.

16 fresh littleneck clams
3 cups water
¼ teaspoon instant dashi granules
2 tablespoons white miso
2 cups gently packed baby spinach
Toasted sesame oil, for drizzling
3 tablespoons thinly sliced green onions (white and
    light green parts)

Wash the clams thoroughly to remove any grit.

In a large lidded saucepan over high heat, bring the water and dashi granules to a boil. Add the clams and return to a boil. Reduce the heat to medium, cover, and cook until the clams open, 4 to 6 minutes. Remove from the heat. Using a slotted spoon, remove the clams from the broth and put in a bowl. Discard any clams that didn't open and let cool.

Into a large heat-proof bowl, pour the broth through a fine-mesh sieve to strain out any grit. Rinse the pan and return the broth to the pan.

Over medium-high heat, bring the broth to a simmer. Reduce the heat to medium-low. Combine the miso with 3 tablespoons of the broth in a small bowl and stir into a smooth paste. Whisk the paste into the simmering broth. Stir in the spinach and cook until wilted, about 1 minute.

Remove the cooked clams from their shells and divide them among four bowls. Ladle the hot broth and spinach over the clams and season with a drop or two of sesame oil. Garnish with green onions.

GROSS CARBS: **5 G**
NET CARBS: **4 G**

Soups and Stews

Tom Yum Soup with Shrimp

Tom yum is a traditional hot and sour Thai soup. If you have access to a specialty Asian supermarket, substitute galangal for ginger and 4 kaffir lime leaves for the lime zest.

1 stalk lemongrass, cut into 1-inch pieces
2¼-inch-thick piece peeled ginger
6 cups reduced-sodium chicken broth
2 jalapeños, sliced
Three 2-inch-wide strips lime zest
1½ cups chopped fresh pineapple
1 cup sliced shiitake mushroom caps
1 tomato, chopped
½ red bell pepper, cut into 1-inch cubes
2 tablespoons fish sauce
1 teaspoon sugar
8 ounces 36- to 30-count raw shrimp, peeled and deveined
¼ cup fresh lime juice
2 green onions, sliced
½ cup chopped fresh cilantro

Gently smash the lemongrass and ginger on a cutting board with the broad side of a knife. Place them in a large lidded saucepan with the broth, jalapeños, and lime zest. Over medium-high heat, bring to a boil, reduce the heat to low, and simmer, covered, for 15 minutes. Strain the broth into a bowl and discard the solids.

Return the broth to the saucepan. Add the pineapple, mushrooms, tomato, bell pepper, fish sauce, and sugar. Over medium-low heat, bring to a simmer and cook, uncovered, for 5 minutes. Add the shrimp and cook until they are pink and cooked through, about 3 minutes. Remove from the heat and stir in the lime juice, green onions, and cilantro.

GROSS CARBS: **15 G**
NET CARBS: **13 G**

Italian Egg Drop Soup

This classic soup is sometimes called stracciatella, which refers to the shredded look the eggs have in the final product. When spinach is in season, you can also add some to the broth.

6 cups chicken broth
3 eggs
¼ cup grated Parmesan
2 tablespoons chopped fresh parsley
Salt and pepper

In a medium saucepan, over moderate heat, bring the broth to a simmer, being careful not to let it boil.

In a small bowl, whisk together the eggs and Parmesan cheese. Slowly pour the egg-cheese mixture into the broth. Wait a minute for the eggs to start to set, then gently stir in the parsley, breaking up the cooked egg. Turn off the heat. Season with salt and pepper. Serve immediately.

GROSS CARBS: **2 G**
NET CARBS: **2 G**

Cioppino

Cioppino may sound Italian, but it is believed to have originated among immigrant fishermen in San Francisco. It is a seafood stew, and the particular ingredients can differ based on taste and what is fresh that day.

5 garlic cloves, minced
2 tablespoons olive oil
One 24-ounce jar tomato-basil pasta sauce
One 8-ounce bottle clam juice
1 cup chicken broth
¼ cup water
1 teaspoon salt
1 teaspoon sugar
1 teaspoon red pepper flakes
1 teaspoon minced fresh basil
1 teaspoon minced fresh thyme
1 pound fresh littleneck clams, scrubbed
1 pound fresh mussels, scrubbed
1 pound 43-50-count raw shrimp, peeled and deveined
1 pound bay scallops
One 6-ounce package baby spinach

In a Dutch oven over medium-high heat, sauté the garlic in the olive oil until tender, 2 to 3 minutes. Add the pasta sauce, clam juice, broth, water, salt, sugar, red pepper flakes, basil, and thyme. Bring to a boil, reduce the heat to medium-low, and simmer uncovered for 10 minutes.

Increase the heat to medium-high. Add the clams, mussels, and shrimp and bring to a boil. Reduce the heat to medium-low, and simmer uncovered for 10 minutes, stirring occasionally.

Stir in the scallops and spinach. Cook for 5 to 7 minutes or until the clams and mussels open, the shrimp turn pink, and the scallops are opaque. Discard any unopened clams or mussels.

GROSS CARBS: **15 G**
NET CARBS: **12 G**

Chicken and Wild Rice Soup

Wild rice has fewer carbs than pasta, so it's substituted for noodles in this chicken soup. If you've never used dried savory before, it's a strong, peppery herb. Substitute dried thyme if you can't find savory.

2 teaspoons canola oil
¼ cup chopped carrot
¼ cup chopped celery
¼ cup chopped onion
¼ cup chopped green bell pepper
¼ cup chopped peeled parsnip
Two 14.5-ounce cans chicken broth
¾ pound bone-in chicken thighs, skin removed
½ teaspoon dried savory
1 garlic clove, minced
⅛ teaspoon salt
⅛ teaspoon pepper
1 cup cooked long-grain and wild rice

In a large lidded saucepan over medium-high heat, heat the oil and sauté the carrot, celery, onion, bell pepper, and parsnip until crisp-tender, about 3 minutes. Add the broth, chicken, savory, garlic, salt, and pepper. Bring to a boil, reduce the heat to low, cover, and simmer until the chicken is cooked through and no longer pink, about 15 minutes.

Remove the chicken from the broth. When cool enough to handle, remove the meat from bones and cut into bite-size pieces. Discard the bones. Add the chicken and rice to the soup, and heat through.

GROSS CARBS: **11 G**
NET CARBS: **12 G**

Chicken Tortilla Soup

Mexican flavors don't have to come wrapped up in a tortilla. This soup is a great way to use leftover chicken breasts or a rotisserie chicken, since it calls for meat that's already been cooked. It's spicy, so top it with something cooling like sour cream.

Cooking spray for saucepan

½ cup chopped red bell pepper

4 cups low-sodium chicken broth

1 tablespoon ground ancho chile powder

2 tablespoons ground cumin

1 teaspoon minced garlic

1 teaspoon chopped fresh cilantro

3 cups cooked shredded boneless skinless chicken breasts

One 10-ounce can Ro-Tel diced tomatoes and green chilies

2 tablespoons canned diced seeded jalapeños

2 cups water

Coat a large saucepan with cooking spray. Over medium-high heat, add the bell pepper and cook until soft, about 3 minutes. Add the chicken broth, ground ancho, cumin, garlic, and cilantro and stir. Add the chicken and simmer. Reduce the heat to medium-low.

In a medium bowl, combine the diced tomatoes, jalapeños, and the water. Purée using an immersion blender, a food processor, or a blender. Add the puréed tomato mixture to the soup and simmer for 20 minutes.

GROSS CARBS: **3.5 G**

NET CARBS: **3 G**

Slow Cooker Beef and Vegetable Soup with Beer

SERVES 6

Beer in a soup? Why not! Use a light brew, like a lager, so the flavor of the beer doesn't overpower the other ingredients.

1 pound lean ground beef
½ cup chopped onion
One 12-ounce bottle beer
One 10.5-ounce can condensed reduced-sodium beef
    broth, undiluted
1½ cups sliced carrots
1¼ cups water
1 cup chopped peeled turnip
½ cup sliced celery
One 4-ounce can mushroom stems and pieces, drained
1 teaspoon salt
1 teaspoon pepper
1 bay leaf
⅛ teaspoon ground allspice

In a large lidded skillet or sauté pan over medium heat, cook the beef and onion until the meat is no longer pink, 8 to 10 minutes. Drain the grease from the pan and transfer the beef and onion mixture to a 5-quart slow cooker. Add the beer, broth, carrots, water, turnip, celery, mushrooms, salt, pepper, bay leaf, and allspice, and stir. Cover and cook on low for 8 hours. Discard the bay leaf and serve.

GROSS CARBS: **8 G**
NET CARBS: **6 G**

Soups and Stews

Classic Chili

Chili recipes can vary hugely—chunks of steak versus ground beef, chicken versus red meat, beans versus no beans. Try this favorite version whenever you want a filling, healthful dinner. Top with cheese, sour cream, and lime wedges.

3 pounds ground beef

3 garlic cloves, minced

¼ cup all-purpose flour

3 tablespoons chili powder

1 tablespoon dried oregano

1 tablespoon ground cumin

Two 14.5-ounce cans beef broth

One 15-ounce can pinto beans, rinsed and drained

1 teaspoon salt

¼ teaspoon pepper

In a Dutch oven over medium heat, cook the beef and garlic until the meat is no longer pink, 8 to 10 minutes. Drain off the fat, leaving the beef in the pot.

In a small bowl, combine the flour, chili powder, oregano, and cumin. Sprinkle the mixture over the meat, stirring until evenly distributed. Add the broth, beans, salt, and pepper.

Bring the chili to a boil, reduce the heat to low, cover, and simmer for up to 2 hours to allow the flavors to blend, stirring occasionally.

GROSS CARBS: **5 G**

NET CARBS: **4 G**

Italian Sausage Soup

SERVES 10

The sausage boosts the protein (and flavor!) of this hearty soup. By breaking up the linguine, you'll ensure people can eat the dish with a spoon.

5 Italian sausage links (4 ounces each), sliced
1 onion, halved and sliced
6 cups water
One 28-ounce can crushed tomatoes
2 zucchini, quartered lengthwise and sliced
½ cup chopped green bell pepper
1 tablespoon beef bouillon granules
½ teaspoon dried basil
½ teaspoon dried oregano
¼ teaspoon pepper
3 ounces uncooked linguine, broken into 2-inch pieces
3 tablespoons grated Parmesan cheese

In a Dutch oven over medium heat, cook the sausage until it's no longer pink, 4 to 5 minutes. Drain off the fat. Add the water, tomatoes, zucchini, bell pepper, bouillon, basil, oregano, and pepper. Bring to a boil and stir in the linguine. Reduce the heat to medium-low, cover, and simmer until the linguine is cooked, 10 to 15 minutes. Sprinkle with the Parmesan and serve.

GROSS CARBS: **15 G**
NET CARBS: **12 G**

Soups and Stews

Jambalaya

SERVES 8

If you've ever been to New Orleans, chances are you've tasted jambalaya. It's a Creole stew that often contains chicken, seafood, sausage, and rice. This recipe leaves out the rice and seafood and adds in some ham for even more meaty flavor.

4 chicken breasts, cubed
2½ teaspoon Cajun seasoning
2 tablespoons butter
1 onion, diced
1 celery stalk, chopped
1 green bell pepper, chopped
3 garlic cloves, minced
Olive oil (if needed)
1 pound ham, cubed
½ pound smoked sausage, cut into bite-size pieces
1 teaspoon Worcestershire sauce
1 teaspoon onion powder
One 15-ounce can diced tomatoes
Two 14-ounce cans beef broth
3 cups water
1 chicken bouillon cube

In a medium bowl, combine the chicken and ½ teaspoon of the Cajun seasoning.

In a Dutch oven over medium-high heat, melt the butter. Brown the chicken on all sides, for 8 to 10 minutes total, then transfer the chicken to a bowl and set aside.

In the same pot, sauté the onion, celery, bell pepper, and garlic until tender (add a little olive oil if the vegetables start to stick), 8 to 10 minutes. Add the ham and sausage and sauté until lightly browned, 3 to 4 minutes. Stir in the Worcestershire sauce, onion powder, tomatoes, broth, water, and bouillon. Bring to a boil, reduce the heat to low, cover, and simmer for 20 minutes. Return the chicken to the pot and heat through for 5 to 6 minutes.

GROSS CARBS: **8 G**
NET CARBS: **7 G**

Salads

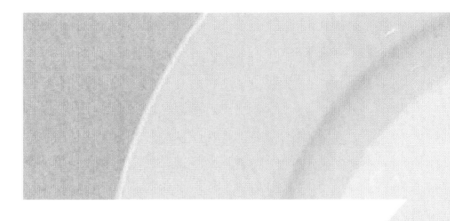

Salads

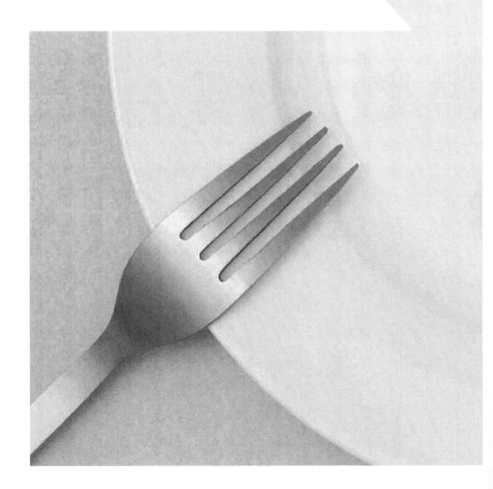

Iceberg Salad with Blue Cheese Dressing

Steakhouses have made this simple salad famous. If you are having company and want to make a statement with the presentation, cut the iceberg lettuce into big wedges and drizzle the dressing over the top.

¼ cup buttermilk
¼ cup crumbled blue cheese
3 tablespoons low-fat sour cream
2 teaspoons lemon juice
Dash of hot sauce
Salt and pepper
10 cups gently packed torn iceberg lettuce leaves

In a large bowl, whisk together the buttermilk, blue cheese, sour cream, lemon juice, and hot sauce. Season with salt and pepper. Add the lettuce and toss to coat.

93

GROSS CARBS: **6 G**
NET CARBS: **3 G**

Salads

Fresh Tomato Salad

SERVES 4

In the summer months, tomatoes are so flavorful that you don't need much to make a great dish. Plus they're packed with antioxidants, vitamin A, and fiber. Heirloom tomatoes are often sold at farmer's markets and, while they may look ugly, are tastier than more mainstream varieties.

1½ pounds tomatoes
Salt and pepper
3 tablespoons balsamic vinegar
2 teaspoons packed light brown sugar
2 tablespoons extra-virgin olive oil
2 teaspoons chopped fresh chives
2 teaspoons chopped fresh basil

Cut the tomatoes into wedges and season with salt and pepper.

In a small skillet or sauté pan over medium heat, cook the balsamic vinegar and brown sugar until the sugar is melted and the mixture is reduced by half, about 3 minutes. Remove from the heat and whisk in the olive oil.

Place the tomatoes on a platter and drizzle the dressing over them. Sprinkle with the chives and basil.

GROSS CARBS: **11 G**
NET CARBS: **9 G**

Low-Carb Cookbook

Broccoli Salad with Tomatoes and Hazelnuts

SERVES 4

Raw broccoli can be a bit tough to eat, but this salad provides two ways around that: The broccoli is sliced as thinly as possible (use a mandoline if you have one), and it marinates in the vinaigrette for 1 hour before serving, which softens and mellows out the vegetable.

1 tablespoon white wine vinegar
Zest of 1 lemon
1 tablespoon fresh lemon juice
2 teaspoons Dijon mustard
1 teaspoon salt
Pinch of pepper
¼ cup extra-virgin olive oil
1 pound broccoli, trimmed and thinly sliced
6 ounces cherry tomatoes, halved
3 ounces coarsely chopped toasted hazelnuts
2 tablespoons sliced fresh basil leaves

In a medium bowl, whisk together the vinegar, lemon zest, lemon juice, Dijon mustard, salt, and pepper. Still whisking, gradually stream in the olive oil. Add the broccoli and toss to coat. Cover and place in the refrigerator for 1 hour to marinate.

Stir in the tomatoes, hazelnuts, and basil. Cover and allow the salad to sit at room temperature for another 15 minutes before serving.

GROSS CARBS: **12 G**
NET CARBS: **6 G**

95

Salads

Mexican Avocado Salad

SERVES 4

The flavors of guacamole star in this simple salad. But unlike the dip, which often comes with high-carb tortilla chips, this salad shines on its own.

2 avocados, peeled, pitted, and sliced
2 tomatoes, seeded and chopped
½ seedless cucumber, chopped
¼ red onion, thinly sliced
1 jalapeño, seeded and minced
3 tablespoons lemon juice
1 garlic clove, minced
A few dashes of hot sauce
1 teaspoon salt
⅓ cup extra-virgin olive oil

On a platter, layer the avocado slices, tomatoes, cucumber, onion, and jalapeño.

In a small bowl, whisk to combine the lemon juice, garlic, hot sauce, and salt. Still whisking, gradually stream in the olive oil. Pour the dressing over the salad and serve.

GROSS CARBS: **14 G**
NET CARBS: **6.5 G**

Grilled Romaine Salad with Citrus Vinaigrette

SERVES 4

It may sound weird to think of grilling a green salad, but for hearty lettuce varieties like romaine, it adds a tasty, smoky, charred flavor. Just make sure to slice the romaine hearts through the core so that the pieces don't fall apart on the grill.

2 romaine hearts, halved lengthwise through the core
4 tablespoons extra-virgin olive oil
Salt and pepper
½ cup crumbled blue cheese
1 navel orange
½ shallot, sliced

Preheat a grill or a grill pan over high heat.

Brush the romaine with 2 tablespoons of the olive oil and season with salt and pepper. Put the romaine on the grill and cook, turning once, until the lettuce begins to wilt and grill marks appear, about 2 minutes. Transfer to a platter and sprinkle with half of the blue cheese.

Over a small bowl, peel the orange and cut away the white pith from the outside. Remove the orange segments by cutting them away from the membrane into the bowl. Squeeze the membrane over the bowl to capture any leftover juice. Drizzle the remaining 2 tablespoons olive oil over the oranges, toss to combine, and season with salt and pepper. Add the shallot to the oranges.

Scatter the oranges and their dressing over the grilled romaine and sprinkle the remaining blue cheese overtop.

GROSS CARBS: **9 G**
NET CARBS: **7 G**

Salads

Caesar Salad
with Mushrooms

SERVES 4

Caesar dressing traditionally has anchovy fillets puréed into it to give a salty, savory flavor. If you don't like the idea of touching anchovy fillets, you can find anchovy paste in the specialty-food section of many grocery stores.

Caesar Dressing
9 canned anchovy fillets, drained and minced
3 tablespoons fresh lemon juice
1½ tablespoons Dijon mustard
2 garlic cloves, minced, plus 4 whole garlic cloves,
    flattened and peeled
½ cup extra-virgin olive oil

1 head romaine lettuce, cut into bite-size pieces
1 head radicchio, cut into bite-size pieces
3 tablespoons olive oil
3 portobello mushrooms, stemmed, caps cut into ⅜-inch-thick slices
Salt and pepper
¼ cup chopped fresh flat-leaf parsley
1⅓ cups coarsely grated Parmesan cheese

To make the Caesar dressing: In a small bowl, whisk together the anchovy fillets, lemon juice, Dijon mustard, and minced garlic. Gradually whisk in the ½ cup olive oil.

In a large bowl, combine the romaine and the radicchio.

In a large heavy skillet or sauté pan over medium heat, heat the 3 tablespoons olive oil. Add the whole garlic cloves and cook until lightly browned, about 4 minutes. Discard the garlic, increase the heat to medium-high, add the mushrooms, and sauté until brown, about 5 minutes. Remove from the heat, season the mushrooms with salt and pepper, and sprinkle with the parsley.

Add the dressing to the lettuces and toss to coat. Mix in the Parmesan. Divide the salad among four plates, top with the mushrooms, and serve immediately.

GROSS CARBS: **10 G**
NET CARBS: **6.5 G**

Summer Salad with Squash, Beets, and Mushrooms

SERVES 6

When it comes to nutritional benefits, it's hard to beat a beet. Beets are high in potassium; magnesium; fiber; phosphorus; iron; vitamins A, B, and C; beta-carotene; and folic acid. Don't just toss the leafy greens—they are great sautéed in olive oil.

1 tablespoon minced shallot
1½ teaspoons Dijon mustard
1½ teaspoons honey
3 tablespoons Champagne vinegar
Salt and pepper
¼ cup olive oil
1 zucchini, cut into 2-inch chunks
1 yellow squash, cut into 2-inch chunks
4 small golden beets, cooked and peeled
3 large white mushrooms
⅓ cup chopped fresh chives

In a small bowl, combine the shallot, Dijon mustard, honey, and vinegar. Season with salt and pepper and whisk in the olive oil.

Thinly slice the zucchini and yellow squash chunks with a mandoline or a vegetable peeler. Thinly slice the beets and mushrooms. In a medium bowl, combine the zucchini, yellow squash, beets, and mushrooms and toss with the vinaigrette. Sprinkle with the chives and season with salt and pepper.

GROSS CARBS: **8 G**
NET CARBS: **6 G**

Salads

Carrot Ribbon Salad with Feta and Dates

SERVES 4

Carrots may be common, but they are still a nutritional superstar. The orange veggie has all the vitamin A your body needs, as well as antioxidants and fiber.

3 carrots

2 tablespoons chopped fresh cilantro

1½ tablespoons olive oil

2 teaspoons honey

½ teaspoon salt

Juice of 1 lime

¼ cup crumbled feta cheese

2 tablespoons chopped toasted almonds

2 tablespoons finely chopped pitted dates

Thinly slice the carrots lengthwise into ribbons using a vegetable peeler or mandoline. In a medium bowl filled with ice water, soak the carrot ribbons until they firm up and curl, about 15 minutes. Drain and pat dry.

In a medium bowl, whisk together the cilantro, olive oil, honey, salt, and lime juice. Add the carrots, feta cheese, almonds, and dates. Toss until combined. Serve immediately or let it sit and marinate in the dressing for a bit before serving.

GROSS CARBS: **9 G**

NET CARBS: **7 G**

Fennel, Ricotta Salata, and Arugula Salad

SERVES 6

Ricotta salata is regular ricotta cheese that's been pressed, salted, and dried. If you can't find it in your grocery store, use Pecorino Romano, Manchego, or some other sheep's milk cheese.

1 shallot, minced
2 tablespoons fresh lemon juice
3 tablespoons extra-virgin olive oil
Salt and pepper
10 cups gently packed arugula
1 fennel bulb, trimmed, halved lengthwise, cored, thinly sliced
3 ounces ricotta salata, shaved into long strips with a
    vegetable peeler

In a small bowl, whisk together the shallot and lemon juice. Gradually whisk in the olive oil and season with salt and pepper. Let stand for 15 minutes.

In a large bowl, combine the arugula and fennel. Toss with enough dressing to coat the salad. Add the shaved ricotta salata, and toss gently. Serve immediately.

GROSS CARBS: **6 G**
NET CARBS: **4.5 G**

Salads

Spinach Salad with Bacon and Egg

SERVES 6

This salad oozes decadence thanks to the warm bacon dressing that's tossed over the spinach just before serving. The spinach will wilt slightly, going perfectly with the eggs, mushrooms, and onion.

7 slices thick-cut bacon
1 small red onion, thinly sliced
8 ounces white button mushrooms, sliced
3 tablespoons red wine vinegar
2 teaspoons sugar
½ teaspoon Dijon mustard
Dash of salt
2 cups gently packed baby spinach
3 hard-boiled eggs, peeled

In a large heavy skillet or sauté pan over medium-high heat, fry the bacon until crispy. Using tongs, transfer the bacon to a plate lined with paper towels and let cool.

Pour the bacon fat into a small bowl and reserve. Wipe the pan with a paper towel. Reduce the heat to medium, add the onion to the pan, and cook until caramelized, 10 to 15 minutes. Remove the onion to a small bowl. Add 1 tablespoon of the reserved bacon fat to the pan, and add the mushrooms. Cook until browned, about 5 minutes, and remove the mushrooms to another small bowl.

Reduce the heat to medium-low, and in a small saucepan, add 3 tablespoons of the reserved bacon fat, the red wine vinegar, sugar, Dijon mustard, and salt. Whisk together and heat thoroughly until bubbly.

Place the spinach in a large salad bowl. Crumble the bacon and arrange on top of the spinach with the onion and mushrooms. Pour the hot dressing over and toss to combine. Crumble the eggs on top and serve.

GROSS CARBS: **7 G**
NET CARBS: **5 G**

Spinach and Fruit Salad with Sesame Dressing

SERVES 6

Fruits and vegetables can mingle in a salad with delicious results. The Asian-style dressing is tart enough to emphasize the sweetness of the fruit. Use whatever stone fruits, tropical fruits, or berries that are in season and available where you live.

2 cups sliced nectarines or peaches
1 cup sliced papaya or mango
½ cup sliced strawberries
½ cup raspberries
¼ cup rice vinegar
1 teaspoon honey
½ teaspoon toasted sesame oil
6 cups gently packed baby spinach
2 tablespoons chopped fresh mint

Salads

In a large bowl, combine the nectarines, papaya, strawberries, and raspberries. Set aside.

In a small bowl, whisk together the rice vinegar, honey, and sesame oil. Pour the vinaigrette over the fruit and toss gently to coat.

Toss the spinach with the dressed fruit and sprinkle with the mint.

GROSS CARBS: **12 G**
NET CARBS: **7 G**

Waldorf Salad

The Waldorf salad was created in New York City at what is now the Waldorf-Astoria Hotel. It traditionally is made with apples, but this version uses jicama. You'll get all the crunch without the carbs.

2 cups diced jicama
½ cup dried cranberries
½ cup chopped walnuts
4 celery stalks, cut into ¼-inch slices
½ cup light mayonnaise
3 tablespoons sugar
1 teaspoon ground cinnamon
1 teaspoon fresh lemon juice
Salt and pepper
12 cups gently packed mixed greens

In a large bowl, combine the jicama, cranberries, walnuts, and celery.

In a small bowl, whisk together the mayonnaise, sugar, cinnamon, and lemon juice. If the dressing seems too thick, add a little water to thin it out.

Pour the dressing over the jicama mixture, and toss to combine well. Refrigerate for 30 minutes to blend the flavors, and then season with salt and pepper. Serve the salad over the mixed greens.

GROSS CARBS: **16 G**
NET CARBS: **13 G**

Low-Carb Cookbook

Spicy Shrimp and Black Bean Salad

SERVES 4

This recipe calls for chipotle chiles in adobo sauce, which are small spicy peppers that have been smoked and canned in a flavor-rich red sauce. They are sold in the Latino-food section of the grocery store. This salad can be made up to 1 day ahead; just cover and refrigerate.

¼ cup cider vinegar

3 tablespoons extra-virgin olive oil

1 tablespoon minced seeded chipotle chile in adobo

1 teaspoon ground cumin

¼ teaspoon salt

1 pound peeled and deveined cooked shrimp, cut into ½-inch pieces

One 15-ounce can black beans, drained and rinsed

1 cup quartered cherry tomatoes

1 large poblano chile, seeded and chopped

¼ cup chopped green onions

¼ cup chopped fresh cilantro

In a large bowl, whisk together the vinegar, olive oil, chipotle chile, cumin, and salt. Add the shrimp, beans, tomatoes, poblano chile, green onions, and cilantro. Toss to combine and serve at room temperature or chilled.

GROSS CARBS: **19 G**

NET CARBS: **13 G**

Herb and Greens Salad with Steak

Mixing fresh herbs in with greens is an easy way to add flavor to a salad. Just go with something leafy, like basil, cilantro, or mint. This recipe calls for hanger steak, but you can substitute skirt steak as long as you grill it for only about 2 minutes per side.

1 shallot, thinly sliced crosswise and separated into rings
¼ cup red wine vinegar
½ cup plus 2 tablespoons extra-virgin olive oil
Salt and pepper
1 eggplant, peeled and cut lengthwise into 1-inch wedges
2 ears of corn
1 pound hanger steak
2 cups gently packed arugula
2 cups packed fresh herb leaves like basil, cilantro, or mint

In a small bowl, combine the shallot and vinegar. Let sit for 5 minutes.

Whisk in ½ cup of the olive oil. Season with salt and pepper. Set aside.

Preheat the grill to medium-high.

Cut each wedge of eggplant in half crosswise. Brush the eggplant and corn ears with the remaining 2 tablespoons olive oil. Season with salt and pepper. Grill, turning often, until the vegetables are tender and charred in spots, 10 to 15 minutes. Let cool and then cut the corn kernels from the cobs.

Season the steak with salt and pepper and grill until medium-rare, 5 to 7 minutes per side. Let rest, then thinly slice against the grain.

In a large bowl, toss the arugula, herbs, eggplant, corn, steak, and vinaigrette and serve.

GROSS CARBS: **19.5 G**
NET CARBS: **14 G**

Fajita Salad

Fajita meat is often served on a bed of grilled bell peppers and onions. This salad takes those ingredients and combines them into a Tex-Mex superstar salad. Feel free to add a low-carb tortilla to make this meal even more hearty.

¼ cup lime juice
¼ cup reduced-sodium chicken broth
1 tablespoon chopped fresh cilantro
2 garlic cloves, minced
1½ teaspoons cornstarch
¾ pounds boneless beef top sirloin steak, cut into
    thin 3-inch strips
½ teaspoon ground cumin
¼ teaspoon salt
¼ teaspoon pepper
Cooking spray for pan
2 small onions, cut into thin wedges
2 green bell peppers, cut into thin strips
1 tablespoon canola oil
8 cups gently packed mixed greens
12 cherry tomatoes, quartered

In a small bowl, combine the lime juice, chicken broth, cilantro, garlic, and cornstarch. Set aside.

Sprinkle the beef with the cumin, salt, and pepper.

Coat an unheated large skillet or sauté pan with cooking spray. Add the onions and bell peppers and stir-fry over medium heat for 3 to 4 minutes or until crisp-tender. Remove the vegetables from pan to a plate.

Add the oil to the pan and add the beef strips. Stir-fry for about 3 minutes or until done to your liking. Push the steak to the side of the pan. Give the lime juice mixture a stir and add it to pan. Cook and stir until thickened and bubbly, then continue cooking for 1 minute more. Add the vegetables to the pan and stir with the meat and lime juice mixture until heated through.

Arrange the mixed greens and tomatoes on a platter. Top with the beef-vegetable mixture.

GROSS CARBS: **13 G**
NET CARBS: **10 G**

Side Dishes

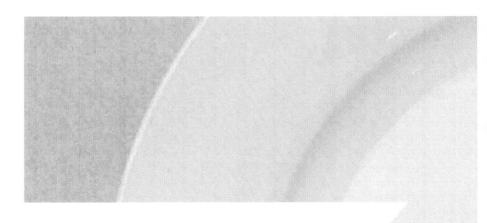

Side Dishes

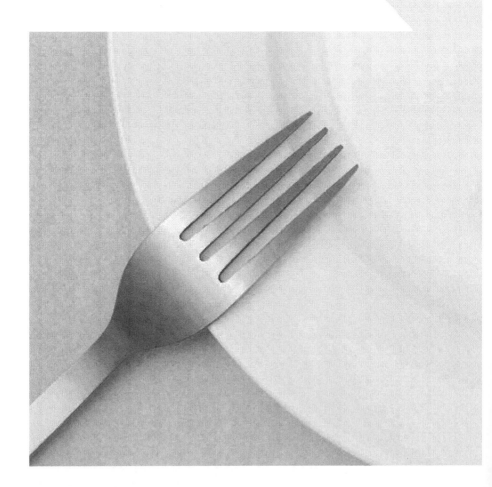

Kale Chips

Kale is a nutrient superstar—packed with vitamin K, vitamin A, vitamin C, and more. But it doesn't just work well in salads or as a sautéed green. It also makes an amazing chip when baked in the oven.

2 bunches kale, thick stems and ribs removed, leaves cut
    into medium pieces
2 tablespoons olive oil
⅛ teaspoon salt
Juice of ½ lime
2 tablespoons grated Parmesan cheese

Preheat the oven to 250°F.

In a large bowl, toss the kale with the olive oil and salt. Spread the kale on a baking sheet and bake until slightly crispy around edges, about 20 minutes. Remove from the oven, drizzle with the lime juice, and sprinkle with the Parmesan cheese. Serve warm.

GROSS CARBS: **14 G**

NET CARBS: **11 G**

111

Side Dishes

Cayenne Pepper Sweet Potato Chips

SERVES 4

The natural sugars in a sweet potato go well with spices like cayenne pepper. More healthful than fried chips, these are still best eaten in moderation when on a low-carb diet.

2 sweet potatoes, peeled
2 tablespoons olive oil
1 teaspoon cayenne pepper
½ teaspoon salt
½ teaspoon black pepper

Preheat the oven to 450°F. Line two baking sheets with parchment paper.

Cut the sweet potatoes into very thin slices.

In a large bowl, mix the olive oil, cayenne pepper, salt, and black pepper. Add the sliced sweet potatoes and toss to coat. Arrange in a single layer on the prepared baking sheets. Bake until crisp, about 10 minutes.

GROSS CARBS: **10 G**
NET CARBS: **8 G**

Classic Coleslaw with a Spicy Twist

SERVES 8

What's a summer picnic without coleslaw? This version skips the heavy mayonnaise in favor of a spicy vinaigrette. Feel free to make it earlier in the day and chill it; just wait until right before serving to add the dressing.

3 carrots, peeled and finely chopped
6 cups gently packed shredded green cabbage
1 red bell pepper, cut into skinny strips
1 red onion, thinly sliced
¾ cup chopped fresh cilantro
⅓ cup fresh lime juice
½ teaspoon ground cumin
1 garlic clove, minced
½ teaspoon hot pepper sauce
½ cup extra-virgin olive oil
Salt and pepper

Over medium-high heat, bring a medium saucepan filled halfway with lightly salted water to a boil and cook the carrots until crisp-tender, about 2 minutes. Drain the carrots, transfer them to a large bowl, and let cool completely. Add the cabbage, bell pepper, onion, and cilantro and toss to mix.

In a medium bowl, whisk together the lime juice, cumin, garlic, and hot pepper sauce. Gradually whisk in olive oil. Season with salt and pepper.

Toss the salad with enough dressing to coat, and season again with salt and pepper if desired. Serve immediately after dressing.

GROSS CARBS: **8 G**
NET CARBS: **5.5 G**

Side Dishes

Mushrooms with Lemon and Pepper

SERVES 4

Mushrooms tend to get added to other dishes—omelets and pizza—or stuffed with a hearty filling. This side dish lets them shine on their own with the simple addition of lemon, pepper, and chives.

1 tablespoon unsalted butter
20 ounces white button mushrooms, sliced
1 tablespoon finely grated lemon zest
¼ teaspoon salt, plus more as needed
¾ teaspoon pepper, plus more as needed
1½ tablespoons minced fresh chives

In a large skillet or sauté pan over medium-high heat, melt the butter. Add the mushrooms and sprinkle with the lemon zest. Cook, undisturbed, until browned, about 2 minutes. Toss with the salt and pepper and continue to cook until the mushrooms are tender but not mushy, 4 to 5 minutes more. Season with salt and pepper. Transfer to a serving dish and sprinkle with the chives. Serve warm.

GROSS CARBS: **5 G**
NET CARBS: **3.5 G**

Mashed Zucchini

SERVES 6

Mashed potatoes are a classic side that can never be replaced, but this version comes close. It's made with mostly zucchini but has other flavorings like green bell pepper and green onion going on, too.

1 green bell pepper, finely chopped
2 tablespoons extra-virgin olive oil
2 tablespoons unsalted butter
1 garlic clove, minced
6 zucchini, halved lengthwise and thinly sliced crosswise
½ cup water
¾ teaspoons salt
½ teaspoon pepper
⅓ cup chopped green onions (green part only)

In a large lidded saucepan over low heat, cook the bell pepper in the olive oil and 1 tablespoon of the butter, stirring occasionally, until the bell pepper is softened, 4 to 6 minutes. Add the garlic and cook for 1 minute, stirring constantly. Add the zucchini, water, salt, and pepper and bring to a boil over medium-high heat. Reduce the heat to medium-low and simmer, covered, for 6 minutes. Remove the lid and simmer until most of the liquid has evaporated and the zucchini is soft, about 6 minutes more. Coarsely mash the zucchini with a potato masher and add the green onions and the remaining 1 tablespoon butter. Stir until the butter is incorporated.

GROSS CARBS: **10 G**
NET CARBS: **6.5 G**

Side Dishes

Creamless Creamed Spinach with Nutmeg Butter

Creamed spinach is a holiday favorite, but it packs an insane calorie and fat punch. This version ditches the heavy cream but still feels festive thanks to the nutmeg and butter. Serve with roasted meat like turkey or roast beef.

1 cup water
4 pounds flat-leaf spinach (about 8 bunches), with
    coarse stems removed
5 tablespoons unsalted butter
1½ teaspoons grated nutmeg
½ teaspoon salt
¼ teaspoon pepper

In a large saucepan over high heat, bring the water to a boil. Add the spinach and cook until completely wilted, about 5 minutes. Drain in a colander, squeezing with back of a spoon to get as much liquid out as you can.

In the same pan over medium heat, melt the butter until foaming subsides. Stir in the nutmeg, salt, and pepper, and then stir in the spinach. Cook, tossing with tongs, until heated through.

GROSS CARBS: **8 G**
NET CARBS: **3 G**

Spinach Pie

SERVES 8

Spanakopita is a popular dish in Greece made with spinach and feta cheese in a flaky pastry crust. This version is slightly altered—no pastry here—but is as salty, creamy, and delicious as the original. It's baked in a pie dish, so slice it into wedges to serve.

Cooking spray for pie pan
20 ounces frozen spinach, thawed, drained, and squeezed dry
3 eggs, lightly beaten
2 teaspoons fresh dill
8 green onions, sliced
⅓ cup grated Parmesan cheese
⅓ cup plain nonfat yogurt
1 tablespoon olive oil
4 ounces feta cheese, crumbled
2 tablespoons fresh lemon juice
½ teaspoon salt
¼ teaspoon pepper

Preheat the oven to 375°F. Coat a glass pie pan with cooking spray.

In a large bowl, combine the spinach, eggs, dill, green onions, Parmesan, yogurt, olive oil, feta, lemon juice, salt, and pepper.

Pour the mixture into the prepared pie pan. Bake for 45 to 50 minutes or until firm and light brown on top. Let cool for 10 minutes before slicing.

GROSS CARBS: **5 G**
NET CARBS: **3 G**

Side Dishes

Brussels Sprouts with Bacon

SERVES 4

Certain flavors just go together, and Brussels sprouts and bacon are one of those pairings. This salty, rich, vegetable side dish is a favorite across the country and goes well with any type of meat.

2 tablespoons olive oil
6 ounces bacon, chopped
½ pound Brussels sprouts, trimmed and halved
¾ teaspoon salt
¾ teaspoon white pepper
¾ cup chicken stock

In a large skillet or sauté pan over medium heat, heat the olive oil until shimmery. Add the bacon and cook until the fat is rendered and bacon is crisp, 5 to 10 minutes. Using a slotted spoon, remove the bacon from the pan and drain on a plate lined with paper towels.

Add the Brussels sprouts, salt, and white pepper to the bacon fat in the pan and sauté over medium heat until lightly browned, about 5 minutes. Add the chicken stock, reduce the heat, and cook until the sprouts are tender, about 15 minutes.

Return the bacon to the pan and heat through.

GROSS CARBS: **9.5 G**
NET CARBS: **6 G**

Snap Peas with Pancetta

SERVES 6

Snap peas come with tough strings running lengthwise on both sides of the pod. To remove them, grab each end of the stem with your fingers and pull the strings.

1½ pounds sugar snap peas, strings removed
1 tablespoon olive oil
2 ounces pancetta, diced
1 leek (white and light green parts only), halved lengthwise
    and sliced
2 garlic cloves, thinly sliced
Pinch of red pepper flakes
½ teaspoon salt, plus more as needed
1 tablespoon white wine vinegar
Pepper

Over medium-high heat, bring a large saucepan of salted water to a boil. Add the snap peas and cook until bright green, about 5 minutes. Drain and run the peas under cold water until they are room temperature. Pat dry.

In a large skillet or sauté pan over medium heat, heat the olive oil. Add the pancetta and cook, stirring, until golden, about 5 minutes. Add the leek, garlic, and red pepper flakes. Cook, stirring, until the leek is soft, about 3 minutes.

Transfer to a large bowl. Add the snap peas and salt and toss. Add the vinegar, season with salt and pepper, and toss again. Serve at room temperature.

GROSS CARBS: **11 G**
NET CARBS: **8 G**

Stuffing with Sausage and Herbs

SERVES 8

Who doesn't love sausage and herb stuffing? This recipe cuts out the stale bread cubes and focuses instead on the delicious herbs and sausage. You don't need to wait for the holidays to make this easy dish!

Cooking spray for baking dish

1 pound pork sausage

¼ cup chopped celery

¼ cup chopped onion

2 eggs, beaten

1 head cauliflower, chopped (about 2 cups)

1 tablespoon chopped fresh parsley

3 tablespoons chopped fresh sage

3 tablespoons chopped fresh thyme

1 tablespoon minced garlic

⅛ teaspoon salt

⅛ teaspoon pepper

Preheat the oven to 350°F. Coat an 8-inch square baking dish with cooking spray.

In a large saucepan over medium heat, brown the sausage. Add the celery and onion and cook until brown; drain the excess fat. Add the eggs, cauliflower, parsley, sage, thyme, garlic, salt, and pepper.

Pour the sausage mixture into the prepared baking dish. Bake until set and brown on top, about 30 minutes.

GROSS CARBS: **3 G**

NET CARBS: **2 G**

Vegetarian Entrées

Stir-Fry with Greens and Walnuts

Portobello Paninis

Zucchini and Tomato Bake

Pizza with Cauliflower Crust

Eggplant, Tomato, and
Feta Napoleons

Eggplant Parmesan

Chile Relleno Lasagna

Ricotta Gnocchi

Spaghetti Squash Alfredo

Roasted Tofu and Asparagus with
Orange and Basil

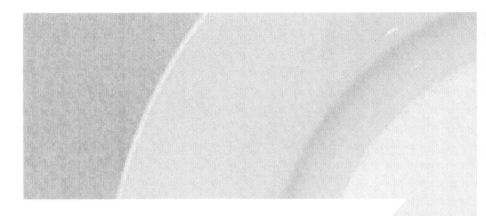

Vegetarian Entrées

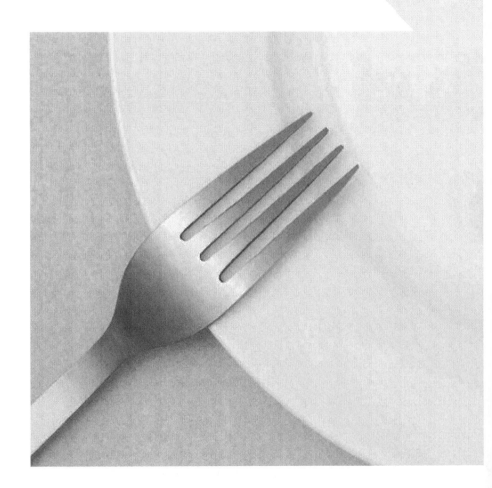

Stir-Fry with Greens and Walnuts

There are so many more edible greens besides spinach and lettuce, and this recipe features two of them: beet greens and mustard greens. Beet greens are the leafy tops of beets and taste a bit sweet, while mustard greens have a sharp, peppery flavor.

1 teaspoon curry powder
¼ teaspoon ground coriander
¼ teaspoon cumin
¼ teaspoon ground cinnamon
½ teaspoon mustard seed
¼ teaspoon cayenne pepper
¼ cup halved walnuts
1 teaspoon olive oil
1 onion, sliced thin
1 garlic clove, sliced
3 bunches spinach, stemmed and coarsely chopped
1 bunch mustard greens, stemmed and coarsely chopped
1 bunch beet greens, coarsely chopped
Salt

Preheat the oven to 350°F.

In a small bowl, combine the curry powder, coriander, cumin, cinnamon, mustard seed, and cayenne. Set aside.

Spread the walnuts in a single layer on a baking sheet and toast until golden brown, about 10 minutes.

In a dry sauté pan over medium-high heat, add half the spice mix and toss to toast, taking care not to burn. Remove from the pan onto a plate.

Add the olive oil to the pan and sauté the onion over medium heat until golden, 10 to 12 minutes. Add the walnuts to the onion and cook for 1 minute more. Season the walnut-onion mixture with the spice mix (both toasted and untoasted portions). Increase the heat to medium-high, and add the spinach, mustard greens, and beet greens to the walnut-onion-spice mixture. Sauté until the greens wilt, about 3 minutes. Season with salt.

GROSS CARBS: **11 G**
NET CARBS: **5 G**

Portobello Paninis

SERVES 2

Pressed grilled sandwiches are always a hit, but this one swaps out the bread and uses meaty portobello mushroom caps instead. The filling here is simple—sun-dried tomatoes and Gorgonzola cheese—but feel free to play around with different flavors. While this recipe makes four sandwiches, they are on the smaller side, so serve each person two.

4 sun-dried tomatoes (dry, not packed in oil)
4 portobello mushrooms, stemmed
¼ cup crumbled Gorgonzola cheese
1 tablespoon plus 1 teaspoon extra-virgin olive oil
Salt and pepper

In a small bowl, cover the sun-dried tomatoes with boiling water and soak for 10 minutes. Drain and roughly chop.

Slice each portobello cap in half horizontally, giving you 8 round mushroom disks. Top 4 of the mushroom cap disks with 1 tablespoon of the chopped tomatoes and 1 tablespoon of the crumbled Gorgonzola. Top with the remaining 4 mushroom disks. Brush the top sides of the sandwiches with half of the olive oil.

Place the mushroom sandwiches in a large nonstick skillet, sauté, or grill pan, oiled-sides down, over medium-high heat, and cook for 2 minutes. Brush the sides that are up with the rest of the olive oil, flip the sandwiches, and cook for 2 minutes more. Season with salt and pepper.

GROSS CARBS: **10 G**

NET CARBS: **7 G**

Zucchini and Tomato Bake

Casseroles don't have to be all meat, pasta, and cheese. This dish is packed with fresh vegetables and loads of spices. Cotija is a hard Mexican cheese that's easy to crumble—it has a flavor that's part feta and part Parmesan.

Cooking spray for coating baking sheet, baking dish, and zucchini
2 pounds zucchini
Salt and pepper
1 teaspoon olive oil
2 garlic cloves, minced
1 jalapeño, seeded and minced
1 teaspoon chili powder
½ teaspoon ground cumin
One 14.5-ounce can no-salt-added fire-roasted diced tomatoes
⅓ cup crumbled Cotija cheese
2 tablespoons chopped fresh cilantro

Preheat the oven broiler. Place an oven rack 5 inches from the broiler. Line a rimmed baking sheet with foil and coat it with cooking spray. Coat an 8-inch square baking dish with cooking spray.

Cut the zucchini on an angle into ½-inch-thick slices. Transfer to the prepared baking sheet. Coat the zucchini with cooking spray and season with salt and pepper. Broil until golden, about 4 minutes, and flip to repeat on the other side. Reduce the oven temperature to 425°F.

In a medium saucepan over medium-high heat, heat the olive oil. Add the garlic and jalapeño and cook until softened, 2 to 3 minutes. Add the chili powder, cumin, and tomatoes. Continue to cook until the tomatoes are soft and the sauce is thickened, about 10 minutes. Remove from the heat, lightly mash with a fork, and season with salt and pepper.

Place half the zucchini slices in the bottom of the prepared baking dish and top with half the tomato sauce. Repeat the layers, then cover with foil and bake until bubbly and hot, about 20 minutes. Remove the foil, sprinkle with the Cojita, and bake for another 10 minutes or until the cheese is melted and lightly browned. Let rest for 10 minutes and sprinkle with the cilantro.

GROSS CARBS: **13 G**
NET CARBS: **10 G**

Pizza with Cauliflower Crust

SERVES 4

Pizza doesn't have to be abandoned completely just because you're eating low-carb. Cauliflower actually makes a tasty crust. If you are craving a crispy crust, place the blanched cauliflower in a strainer over another bowl in the refrigerator overnight to let any excess water drain out.

Cooking spray for coating pizza pan and crust
1 cup tomato sauce
1 garlic clove, chopped
¼ teaspoon dried basil
½ bay leaf
¼ teaspoon dried oregano
¼ teaspoon dried thyme
24 ounces cauliflower, cut into florets
½ cup grated Parmesan cheese
2 egg whites
1 teaspoon baking powder
Salt and pepper
1 cup shredded part-skim mozzarella cheese

Preheat the oven to 400°F. Coat a round pizza pan with cooking spray.

In a small saucepan over medium-high heat, add the tomato sauce, garlic, basil, bay leaf, oregano, and thyme. Bring to a simmer, reduce the heat to low, and lightly simmer for 10 minutes. Remove from the heat.

Fill a medium saucepan halfway with water, and bring it to a boil. Blanch the cauliflower for 5 to 7 minutes or until soft and a floret can be crushed with the tines of a fork. Strain the cauliflower and place it in an ice bath to stop cooking. When cooled, strain the cauliflower.

In a food processor, chop the cauliflower until it resembles coarse meal. Place the cauliflower in a large mixing bowl. Add the Parmesan, egg whites, and baking powder and season with salt and pepper.

Press the cauliflower mixture into the prepared pizza pan. Coat the top of the mixture with cooking spray and bake for 30 minutes. Turn on the broiler, place an oven rack about 5 inches below the broiler, and broil the cauliflower crust until the top is browned, 2 to 3 minutes.

Top the crust with the tomato sauce and the mozzarella, and bake until the cheese is melted, about 15 minutes.

GROSS CARBS: **14 G**
NET CARBS: **12 G**

Eggplant, Tomato, and Feta Napoleons

A Napoleon is any dish that consists of layers of ingredients stacked on top of each other. While the term is often used to describe desserts, it can also be applied to savory items, like this recipe.

3 tablespoons red wine vinegar
2 teaspoons minced fresh rosemary
Salt and pepper
¼ cup plus 2 tablespoons olive oil
1 eggplant
2 tomatoes
¼ pound feta cheese, crumbled

Prepare a grill so that the temperature on one side is hot and the other side is medium-low.

In a small bowl, whisk together the vinegar and rosemary and season with salt and pepper. Slowly whisk in the olive oil.

Peel the eggplant and cut it into 12 slices. Cut each tomato crosswise into 4 slices (so you have 8 slices total). Brush the eggplant and tomato slices generously with the dressing.

Grill the eggplant on the hot side until just cooked through, 2 to 3 minutes per side, brushing with more of the dressing halfway through. Grill the tomato slices for 1 minute per side on the hot side of the grill.

Create 4 stacks of vegetables on the cooler side of the grill. Start with a slice of eggplant, then tomato, then some feta, then another slice of eggplant and tomato and more feta. Cover the grill and cook the stacks for 3 to 5 minutes more or until the feta melts.

GROSS CARBS: **11 G**
NET CARBS: **6 G**

Eggplant Parmesan

This version of the classic eggplant Parmesan doesn't use breading, which cuts way down on the carbs. Reduce the carb count even more by finding no-sugar-added marinara sauce.

Cooking spray for baking dish
1½ pounds eggplant, peeled
1 cup shredded Parmesan cheese
2 cups shredded mozzarella cheese
1½ cups marinara sauce
2 teaspoons Italian seasoning
2 teaspoons dried oregano
2 teaspoons dried basil

Preheat the oven to 375°F. Coat a medium baking dish with cooking spray.

Cut the eggplant into ¼-inch-thick slices and place half the eggplant on the bottom of the prepared baking dish. Top with ½ cup of the Parmesan, ¾ cup of the mozzarella, and ¾ cup of the marinara sauce. Sprinkle with 1 teaspoon of the Italian seasoning, 1 teaspoon of the oregano, and 1 teaspoon of the basil. Repeat the layers, and cover the dish with aluminum foil. Bake until the eggplant is tender, approximately 40 minutes. Uncover and top with the remaining ½ cup mozzarella and bake until the cheese is melted, 5 minutes more.

GROSS CARBS: **18 G**
NET CARBS: **13 G**

Vegetarian Entrées

Chile Relleno Lasagna

SERVES 5

Chile rellenos are stuffed chiles—a favorite of Mexican cuisine. Instead of going through the work of stuffing each chile, for this recipe, you layer the flavors and bake the dish in the oven.

Cooking spray for baking dish
One 27-ounce can whole green chiles
4 cups packaged shredded Mexican cheese blend
One 6-ounce can sliced pitted black olives
5 eggs
½ cup milk
½ teaspoon ground cumin
½ teaspoon chili powder

Preheat the oven to 375°F. Coat a 9-by-11-inch baking dish with cooking spray.

Drain the chiles and layer half of them in the bottom of the prepared baking dish. Spread 2 cups of the cheese over them and then half of the black olives. Repeat the layers.

In a medium bowl, beat the eggs. Add the milk, cumin, and chili powder. Mix well, and pour over the chiles.

Cover with foil and bake for 15 minutes. Remove the foil and cook until browned and bubbling, 15 to 25 more minutes.

GROSS CARBS: **5 G**
NET CARBS: **4 G**

Ricotta Gnocchi

SERVES 6

Gnocchi is a decadent potato and flour pasta that obviously is less than low-carb-friendly. In this version, the dumplings are made with mostly ricotta cheese and the flour just gets dusted on the outside instead of mixed in. Serve with your favorite pasta sauce, shavings of Parmesan, or butter sage sauce.

1 pound fresh ricotta cheese
1 egg, lightly beaten
¼ cup grated Parmesan cheese
Salt
Flour for coating

Line a cookie sheet with parchment paper.

In a large bowl, whip the ricotta with a fork to break up the curds. Add the egg and stir well. Add the Parmesan and mix well. Season with salt.

Sprinkle some flour in a large shallow dish. Using two teaspoons, make oval-shaped gnocchi, using about ½ teaspoon of dough at a time. Drop each gnocchi into the flour (don't let them touch or they'll stick to each other). Repeat, to make 6 gnocchi. Coat them lightly with flour by rolling the dish. Carefully brush excess flour off the gnocchi and place them on the prepared cookie sheet. Repeat this process until all the gnocchi are made. Refrigerate the gnocchi for 2 hours or until firm.

To cook the gnocchi, bring a large saucepan of salted boiling water to a simmer. Add the gnocchi and cook until they float to the top, 7 to 9 minutes. Remove with a slotted spoon.

GROSS CARBS: **2.5 G**
NET CARBS: **2.5 G**

Spaghetti Squash Alfredo

SERVES 4

Alfredo sauce, a creamy cheesy choice, is often served over fettuccine. Skip the noodles and use spaghetti squash, which looks like pasta and does a fabulous job of carrying the sauce.

1 spaghetti squash
1 cup low-fat sour cream
½ cup shredded mozzarella cheese
¼ cup grated Parmesan cheese
¼ teaspoon salt
¼ teaspoon pepper

Preheat the oven to 375°F.

Cut the squash in half and scoop out and discard the seeds. Place the squash halves cut-side up on a baking sheet, and bake until a fork goes in easily, 45 to 50 minutes. Take out of the oven, and let cool. Scrape the squash into strands using a fork, and place in a medium bowl.

In a medium saucepan over medium-low heat, combine the sour cream, mozzarella, Parmesan, salt, and pepper. Cook, whisking until smooth and creamy, until heated through, 5 minutes. Add the spaghetti squash to the sauce and gently toss to combine.

GROSS CARBS: **18 G**
NET CARBS: **14.5 G**

Roasted Tofu and Asparagus with Orange and Basil

You may know miso from the soup you get at sushi restaurants, but the thought of cooking with it can be a little intimidating. It shouldn't be! Miso is a simple-to-use paste that comes in different varieties. This recipe uses red miso, which can be found near the tofu in the refrigerated section of most grocery stores.

Cooking spray for baking sheet
One 14-ounce package extra-firm water-packed tofu, drained
2 tablespoons red miso
2 tablespoons balsamic vinegar
4 teaspoons olive oil
1 pound asparagus, ends trimmed, cut into 1-inch pieces
3 tablespoons chopped fresh basil
1 teaspoon freshly grated orange zest
¼ cup orange juice
¼ teaspoon salt

Preheat the oven to 450°F. Coat a large rimmed baking sheet with cooking spray.

Pat the tofu dry and cut it into ½-inch cubes.

In a large bowl, whisk together 1 tablespoon of the miso, 1 tablespoon of the vinegar, and 2 teaspoons of the olive oil until smooth. Add the tofu cubes and gently toss to coat. Spread the tofu in an even layer on the prepared baking sheet and roast for 15 minutes.

Gently toss the asparagus pieces with the tofu in the baking sheet and roast for 8 to 10 minutes more or until the tofu is golden brown and the asparagus is tender.

In a large bowl, whisk the remaining 1 tablespoon miso, 1 tablespoon vinegar, and 2 teaspoons olive oil with the basil, orange zest, orange juice, and salt until smooth. Spoon the roasted tofu and asparagus into the bowl, toss with the sauce, and serve.

GROSS CARBS: **10 G**
NET CARBS: **6 G**

Fish and Seafood

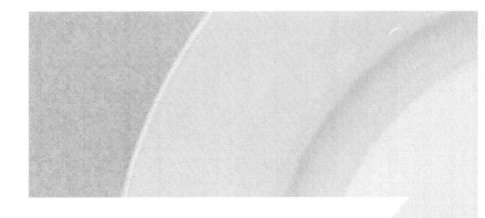

Fish and Seafood

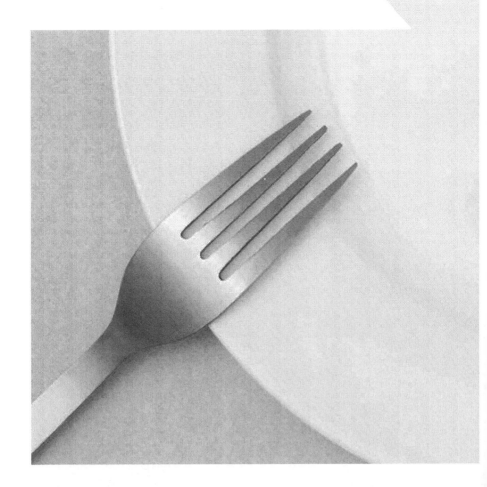

Beer-Steamed Mussels

SERVES 4

Mussels are delicious, inexpensive seafood that cook up quickly. If you notice any are open before you cook them, toss them. And after you're done steaming them, throw out any that stayed shut—that means they're dead and shouldn't be eaten.

2 tablespoons olive oil
1 onion, finely chopped
4 garlic cloves, thinly sliced
One 12-ounce bottle lager beer
¼ teaspoon salt
¼ teaspoon pepper
4 pounds fresh mussels, scrubbed
½ cup chopped parsley

In a heavy 5- or 6-quart lidded pot over medium heat, heat the olive oil, and cook the onion and garlic, until fragrant and slightly softened, about 3 minutes. Add the beer, salt, and pepper and bring to a boil.

Increase the heat to medium-high, add the mussels, and cook, covered, until most of mussels are opened, 6 to 8 minutes. Stir in the parsley and serve.

GROSS CARBS: **17 G**
NET CARBS: **17 G**

Ginger-Roasted Shrimp

SERVES 2

If you find it hard to find deveined shrimp, you can devein them yourself by cutting along the back of the shrimp with kitchen shears and removing the vein. Cook up some spinach, asparagus, or green beans to go alongside this dish.

¼ cup canola oil
¼ cup finely chopped green onions
¼ cup chopped fresh cilantro
2 garlic cloves, minced
1 tablespoon seasoned rice vinegar
2 teaspoons grated peeled fresh ginger
1 teaspoon sesame oil
Salt and pepper
Ten 26- to 30-count raw shrimp, deveined, with shells on
4 ounces oyster mushrooms

Preheat the oven to 500°F.

In a medium bowl, combine the canola oil, green onions, cilantro, garlic, vinegar, ginger, and sesame oil. Season with salt and pepper.

Pull off the legs from the shrimp. Rub some of the oil-spice mixture on the shrimp, making sure to get the undersides coated. Arrange in a single layer on a baking sheet.

Add the mushrooms to the remaining oil-spice mixture in the bowl and toss to coat. Arrange the mushrooms on the baking sheet with the shrimp. Roast until the shrimp are opaque in the center and the mushrooms are tender, about 7 minutes.

GROSS CARBS: **11 G**
NET CARBS: **9 G**

Thai Shrimp Stir-Fry

When you order takeout, you never really know what you're getting in terms of carbohydrates. This dish is just as good as any you'd find at a Thai restaurant, and you'll know you're sticking to your eating plan. Remove the seeds from the jalapeño if you don't like a lot of heat.

2 tablespoons reduced-sodium soy sauce
1 tablespoon water
2 teaspoons fish sauce
4 teaspoons packed light brown sugar
3 tablespoons peanut oil
3 garlic cloves, minced
1 tablespoon grated peeled fresh ginger
½ teaspoon red pepper flakes
1 pound large raw shrimp, peeled and deveined
½ red onion, cut into 1-inch dice
1 yellow bell pepper, seeded and cut into 1-inch dice
1 jalapeño, thinly sliced into rounds
2 cups cherry tomatoes, halved
¾ cup torn fresh basil leaves
¼ cup torn fresh mint leaves
2 tablespoons lime juice

In a small bowl, combine the soy sauce, water, fish sauce, and brown sugar.

In a large nonstick skillet or sauté pan over medium-high heat, heat the oil. Add the garlic, ginger, and red pepper flakes and cook until fragrant, about 30 seconds. Add the shrimp and stir-fry until pink but still translucent in the middle, about 2 minutes. Using a slotted spoon, transfer the shrimp to a medium bowl.

Add the onion, bell pepper, and jalapeño to the pan and stir-fry until lightly browned, about 2 minutes. Return the shrimp to the pan along with the soy sauce mixture. Bring to a boil and stir-fry until the sauce glazes the shrimp, about 1 minute more. Add the tomatoes and stir until coated with sauce, about 15 seconds. Remove the pan from heat, and stir in the basil, mint, and lime juice.

GROSS CARBS: **13 G**
NET CARBS: **11 G**

Crab Cakes

SERVES 6

Often associated with the state of Maryland, crab cakes are a delicious way to eat lump crabmeat without having to shell the crabs. Chill these for 1 hour in the fridge before frying and they'll hold together better in the skillet. The recipe calls for fresh bread crumbs, which are made by tearing the crust off sandwich bread and processing in a food processor until fine.

1½ cups fresh white bread crumbs (from about 5 pieces of bread)
12 ounces fresh or canned crabmeat (about 2 cups)
2 tablespoons chopped fresh dill
2 tablespoons chopped fresh flat-leaf parsley
1 green onion, thinly sliced
2 teaspoons Old Bay Seasoning
¼ teaspoon salt
⅛ teaspoon pepper
1 egg
3 tablespoons light mayonnaise
1 tablespoon lemon juice
2 teaspoons Dijon mustard
⅓ cup unseasoned dry bread crumbs
Cooking spray for baking sheet
4 teaspoons olive oil

Line a baking sheet with plastic wrap.

In a large bowl, combine the fresh bread crumbs and crabmeat. Add the dill, parsley, green onion, Old Bay Seasoning, salt, and pepper. Toss to mix well.

In a small bowl, whisk together the egg, mayonnaise, lemon juice, and Dijon mustard until smooth. Drizzle over the crab mixture and stir well. Using your hands, form the mixture into 6 patties (about ½ cup of crab mixture each). Dredge the patties in the dry bread crumbs and place on the baking sheet lined with plastic wrap. Cover with plastic wrap and refrigerate for 1 hour.

Preheat the oven to 450°F. Coat a baking sheet with cooking spray.

In a large skillet or sauté pan over medium heat, heat 2 teaspoons of the olive oil. Add 3 crab cakes and cook until golden on the underside, 2 to 3 minutes. Place the crab cakes on the prepared baking sheet. Add the remaining 2 teaspoons olive oil to the pan and repeat with remaining crab cakes. Transfer the baking sheet to the oven and bake until golden on the top side and heated through, 15 to 20 minutes.

GROSS CARBS: **20 G**
NET CARBS: **19 G**

Cod and Asparagus en Papillote

The phrase en papillote *means that you are cooking something wrapped up in a piece of paper. In this recipe, each serving is wrapped individually, so you'll need four 15-by-15-inch squares of parchment paper.*

2 tablespoons butter cut into 4 pieces, plus more for the
    parchment paper
Four 6-ounce cod fillets
Salt and pepper
12 fresh tarragon leaves
1 pound asparagus, ends trimmed and cut into 1½-inch pieces
4 tablespoons orange juice

Preheat the oven to 400°F. Generously butter half of each parchment square.

Top the buttered half of each parchment square with 1 fish fillet. Season with salt and pepper and top each fillet with 3 tarragon leaves and 1 piece of butter.

Arrange the asparagus around the fish and pour 1 tablespoon orange juice over each. Fold the parchment over the fish and asparagus, folding the edges tightly to seal and enclose the filling.

Place 2 packets on each of two baking sheets. Bake for 17 minutes. To serve, place a cooked packet on a plate and let your guest open it at the table.

GROSS CARBS: **6 G**

NET CARBS: **4 G**

Fish Tacos with Mango Salsa

These fish tacos get the low-carb treatment by swapping out flour tortillas for big pieces of butter lettuce. If you can't find butter lettuce, look for Bibb or Boston—they are almost the same thing.

2 tablespoons olive oil
1 tablespoon fresh lime juice
½ teaspoon chili powder
1 jalapeño, seeded and diced
4 halibut fillets
2 plum tomatoes, diced
1 mango, peeled and diced
1 onion, chopped
Juice from 1 lime
1 avocado, peeled and diced
8 butter lettuce leaves

In a bowl, whisk together the olive oil, lime juice, chili powder, and jalapeño. Add the halibut fillets and let marinate for 30 minutes.

Preheat the grill to high heat.

In a medium bowl, combine the tomatoes, mango, onion, lime juice, and avocado. Set aside.

Grill the fish until cooked through, 3 to 4 minutes per side. Cut the fish into bite-size pieces and serve with lettuce wraps and the mango salsa.

GROSS CARBS: **15 G**
NET CARBS: **11 G**

Bacon-Wrapped Halibut

Wrapping bacon around anything instantly makes it better. This recipe proves that by taking marinated halibut and wrapping it up in the cured pork. Partially cooking the bacon beforehand ensures that it finishes cooking at the same time as the fish.

½ cup lime juice
½ cup finely chopped onion
2 tablespoons olive oil
2 tablespoons chopped seeded jalapeño
2 tablespoons chopped fresh cilantro
1 teaspoon salt
¼ teaspoon pepper
Four 6- to 8-ounce halibut steaks
8 slices bacon

In a shallow glass dish, combine the lime juice, onion, olive oil, jalapeño, cilantro, salt, and pepper. Add the halibut steaks to the marinade and set aside to marinate for 10 minutes, turning once.

Arrange the bacon in a single layer between paper towels. Microwave for 3 to 4 minutes or until translucent. Wrap 2 slices of bacon around the tops and sides of each halibut steak (leaving the bottom bare), securing the ends with toothpicks.

Heat an outdoor grill or stovetop grill pan to medium-high.

Place the halibut steaks on the grill, bacon-side down. Grill for 4 to 6 minutes per side or until the fish flakes easily with a fork. Remove the toothpicks and serve.

GROSS CARBS: **3 G**
NET CARBS: **3 G**

Tuna Steaks with Cilantro Garlic Sauce

Tuna doesn't just come in a can—you can buy lean and delicious tuna steaks at the seafood counter. This recipe lets the flavor of the fish shine through with a very simple sauce made from cilantro, lime, garlic, and jalapeño.

4 garlic cloves, minced
6 tablespoons olive oil
1 jalapeño, halved lengthwise, seeded, and thinly sliced
½ cup coarsely chopped fresh cilantro
Juice of 4 limes
1 teaspoon salt, plus more as needed
Two 12-ounce tuna steaks
Pepper

Heat an outdoor grill or stovetop grill pan to medium-high.

In a medium bowl, combine the garlic and 4 tablespoons of the olive oil. Cover loosely with plastic wrap and microwave until the garlic is soft and aromatic, about 2 minutes. Stir the jalapeño, cilantro, lime juice, and salt into the hot oil. Set aside to cool.

Brush the tuna steaks with the remaining 2 tablespoons olive oil and season with salt and pepper. Grill, turning once, until grill marks are seared into the fish (3 to 5 minutes per side for medium-rare, 4 to 6 minutes per side for medium-well). Let the tuna rest for 5 minutes, then slice each steak in half crosswise, drizzle with sauce, and serve.

GROSS CARBS: **1 G**
NET CARBS: **1 G**

Fish and Seafood

Salmon with Miso and Ginger

SERVES 4

In this recipe, salmon gets an Asian treatment. The finished dish can be drizzled with yuzu juice if you'd like—a liquid made from a sour Japanese citrus fruit that tastes like a mix between a grapefruit and a lime. Most specialty grocery stores carry yuzu juice in bottles.

¼ cup white miso
¼ cup mirin
2 tablespoons unseasoned rice vinegar
3 tablespoons reduced-sodium soy sauce
2 tablespoons minced green onions
1½ tablespoons minced peeled fresh ginger
2 teaspoons toasted sesame oil
Four 8-ounce salmon fillets
Salt and pepper

In a small bowl, whisk together the miso, mirin, vinegar, soy sauce, green onions, ginger, and sesame oil.

Place the salmon in a baking dish, pour the marinade over it, and turn to coat. Cover and refrigerate for 30 minutes.

Heat an outdoor grill or stovetop grill pan to high.

Remove the fish from the marinade and season with salt and pepper. Grill the salmon, skin-side down, covered, until golden brown and a crust has formed, 3 to 4 minutes. Turn the salmon over and grill for another 3 to 4 minutes.

GROSS CARBS: **6 G**
NET CARBS: **4.5 G**

Brown Sugar and Mustard Grilled Salmon

When exposed to heat, brown sugar melts and caramelizes, turning into an amazing glaze for grilled fish. Instead of using 8 fillets, you can pick up a few longer sides of salmon—they just might be harder to turn over once they're on the grill.

3 tablespoons packed light brown sugar
1 tablespoon honey
2 tablespoons butter
¼ cup Dijon mustard
2 tablespoons reduced-sodium soy sauce
2 tablespoons olive oil
1 tablespoon finely grated peeled ginger
Eight 6-ounce salmon fillets
2 tablespoons vegetable oil
Salt and pepper

In a small sauté pan over medium-high heat, melt the brown sugar, honey, and butter. Remove from the heat and whisk in the Dijon mustard, soy sauce, olive oil, and ginger. Let cool.

Preheat an outdoor grill or stovetop grill pan to medium heat.

Brush the salmon fillets with the vegetable oil and season with salt and pepper. Place the salmon skin-side down on the grill. Coat the exposed salmon side with the brown sugar mixture. Grill for 6 to 8 minutes total, turning over after 5 to 6 minutes.

GROSS CARBS: **4 G**
NET CARBS: **4 G**

Poultry, Pork, and Beef

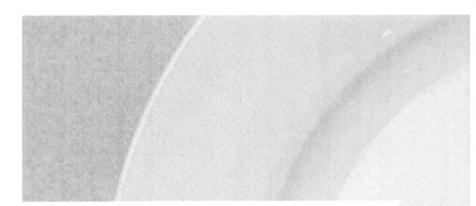

Poultry, Pork, and Beef

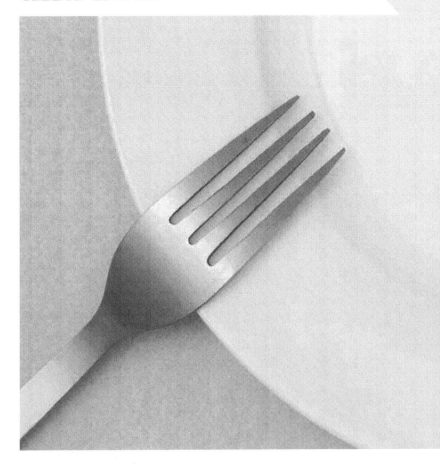

Chicken with Blackening Spices and Fresh Fruit Salsa

This dish gets its spice from two different places: sambal and a blackening spice mix. Sambal is a jarred red sauce that has a chile base and can be picked up in Asian aisles of grocery stores. Blackening spices, which are often with the regular spices, are often used with Cajun food and are a mix of paprika, oregano, thyme, cayenne pepper, black pepper, white pepper, and garlic powder.

2 teaspoons rice wine vinegar
Juice of 2 lemons
1 teaspoon sugar
1 tablespoon sambal
2 cups raspberries
½ cup canned diced pineapple
¼ cup diced strawberries
1 kiwi, peeled and diced
2 tablespoons julienned red onion
1 tablespoon chopped fresh cilantro
1 teaspoon minced fresh mint
6 skinless chicken breasts
2 tablespoons blackening spices
1 tablespoon grapeseed oil

In a medium bowl, whisk together the vinegar, lemon juice, sugar, and sambal. Add the raspberries, pineapple, strawberries, kiwi, red onion, cilantro, and mint and toss to combine. Cover and refrigerate for 20 to 30 minutes.

Coat the chicken breasts with the blackening spices.

In a large heavy lidded skillet or sauté pan over medium-high heat, add the grapeseed oil and allow it to heat. Add the chicken, cover, and cook for 4 minutes, then reduce the heat to medium-low and turn the chicken over. Cover and cook until the chicken has reached an internal temperature of 165°F, 13 to 15 minutes more.

Serve the chicken topped with the fruit salsa.

GROSS CARBS: **12 G**
NET CARBS: **8 G**

Chicken with 40 Cloves of Garlic

SERVES 6

It sounds like a lot, but as the garlic roasts, it loses its intensity and becomes beautifully rich and mellow. Peeling all those garlic cloves can get a little tedious, but it's easier if you soak the cloves in water for 5 minutes beforehand.

1 whole chicken, cut into 8 pieces
Salt and pepper
½ cup plus 2 tablespoons olive oil
10 sprigs fresh thyme
40 garlic cloves, peeled

Preheat the oven to 350°F.

Season the chicken with salt and pepper and toss with 2 tablespoons of the olive oil.

Heat a large lidded skillet or sauté pan over high heat and brown chicken on both sides. Remove the pan from the heat, add the remaining ½ cup olive oil, the thyme, and garlic cloves. Cover and bake in the preheated oven for 1½ hours.

Remove the chicken from the oven, let rest for 5 to 10 minutes, cut the meat off the bone, and serve.

GROSS CARBS: **6 G**
NET CARBS: **5.5 G**

Chicken Paprikash

This Hungarian dish gets its name from all the paprika in it. While there are different kinds of paprika available, see if you can find a sweet version (as opposed to sharp). You can find it in specialty spice shops.

4 skinless boneless chicken breasts, cut crosswise
    into ½-inch-wide strips
8 teaspoons paprika, preferably Hungarian sweet
Salt and pepper
3 tablespoons butter
1 cup chopped onion
2 large plum tomatoes, seeded and chopped
2 cups low-sodium chicken broth
½ cup low-fat sour cream

Season the chicken with 2 teaspoons of the paprika. Season with salt and pepper.

In a large skillet or sauté pan over medium-high heat, melt 2 tablespoons of the butter. Add the chicken and sauté until cooked through, about 3 minutes. Using a slotted spoon, transfer the chicken to a plate.

Add the remaining 1 tablespoon butter to the pan. Add the onion and sauté until it begins to soften, about 3 minutes. Add the remaining 6 teaspoons paprika, and stir for 10 seconds. Add the tomatoes and stir for 1 minute. Add the broth. Increase the heat to high and boil until the sauce thickens, about 5 minutes. Mix in the chicken and any collected juices on the plate. Reduce the heat to low, add the sour cream, and stir until heated through. Season with salt and pepper.

GROSS CARBS: **9.5 G**
NET CARBS: **6.5 G**

Eastern Carolina-Style Barbecued Chicken

SERVES 4

When most people think about barbecue sauce, they think of the sweet, tomato-based version found at most BBQ joints. But in the eastern part of North Carolina, the sauce is actually much more tart and vinegar-based. The good news is that without all that sugar, the carb count is pretty low.

1¼ cups cider vinegar

4 teaspoons chili powder

2½ teaspoons salt

1½ teaspoons sugar

1 teaspoon cayenne pepper

1 teaspoon dry mustard

1 teaspoon paprika

1 teaspoon black pepper

½ teaspoon ground cumin

4 skinless boneless chicken breasts

Preheat the grill to medium-high heat.

In a small bowl, whisk together the vinegar, chili powder, salt, sugar, cayenne, mustard, paprika, pepper, and cumin.

Arrange the chicken in a shallow glass dish and spoon ¼ cup of the sauce over it. Turn the chicken pieces to coat evenly. Let stand for 10 to 20 minutes, turning the chicken occasionally.

Grill the chicken until cooked through, basting occasionally with another ¼ cup sauce, about 5 minutes per side. Serve with the remaining sauce.

GROSS CARBS: **8 G**

NET CARBS: **7 G**

Turkey Meatloaf

When it comes to comfort food, nothing beats meatloaf. This version, made with turkey instead of meat and with oats instead of bread crumbs, is a tasty improvement on the original.

¾ cup quick-cooking oats
½ cup skim milk
1 onion
2 pounds ground turkey breast
½ cup seeded chopped red bell pepper
2 eggs, beaten
2 teaspoons Worcestershire sauce
¼ cup ketchup
½ teaspoon salt
Pepper
One 8-ounce can tomato sauce

Preheat the oven to 350°F.

In a small bowl, stir together the oats and milk and let sit.

Thinly slice one-quarter of the onion and set aside. Finely chop the remaining onion.

In a large bowl, combine the turkey, oats and milk, chopped onion, bell pepper, eggs, Worcestershire sauce, ketchup, and salt, and season with pepper. Mix with your hands until just combined.

Transfer the mixture to a 9-by-13-inch baking dish and shape into a loaf about 5 inches wide and 2 inches high. Pour the tomato sauce over the meatloaf and sprinkle with the sliced onions.

Bake for about 1 hour or until an instant-read thermometer registers 160°F. Let rest for 10 to 15 minutes before slicing.

GROSS CARBS: **13 G**
NET CARBS: **11 G**

Pork Lettuce Wraps

Many Asian restaurants offer lettuce wraps—delicious ground meat filling in a piece of iceberg lettuce. This one has all the great flavors you'd find when eating out, with carrots for crunch and red pepper flakes adding heat.

1 pound ground pork
1 onion, thinly sliced
2 tablespoons grated fresh ginger
1 garlic clove, minced
2 cups coleslaw mix with carrots
1 teaspoon sesame oil
3 tablespoons reduced-sodium soy sauce
2 tablespoons fresh lime juice
1 tablespoon sugar
2 teaspoons ground coriander
½ teaspoon red pepper flakes
8 iceberg lettuce leaves

In a large skillet or sauté pan over medium-high heat, brown the pork and onion. Keeping the pork in the pan, drain off the fat. Add the ginger, garlic, and coleslaw mix. Stir-fry until the vegetables have wilted, about 2 minutes. In a small bowl, combine the sesame oil, soy sauce, lime juice, sugar, coriander, and red pepper flakes, and add to the pan. Stir and cook for 1 minute. Spoon into the lettuce leaves and roll up to eat.

GROSS CARBS: **11 G**
NET CARBS: **10 G**

Asian-Style Grilled Pork Chops

SERVES 4

This recipe combines classic flavors like soy sauce, sesame oil, and ginger with black bean garlic sauce, which you can find in jars in the Asian-food aisle of the grocery store. Any vegetable works well with this dish, but here the pork is paired with bok choy to keep the Asian theme going.

⅓ cup black bean garlic sauce
3 garlic cloves, minced
1½ tablespoons reduced-sodium soy sauce
1½ tablespoons toasted sesame oil
1 tablespoon lime juice
1 tablespoon peeled, minced fresh ginger
4 boneless center-cut pork chops
4 baby bok choy, halved lengthwise
2 tablespoons chopped fresh cilantro

Preheat the grill to medium-high heat.

In a shallow dish, whisk together the black bean sauce, garlic, soy sauce, sesame oil, lime juice, and ginger. Reserve 2 tablespoons of the marinade in a small bowl. Add the pork chops to the remaining marinade and let stand for 20 minutes.

Remove the pork from the marinade, and discard the marinade. Grill the pork until cooked through and a meat thermometer inserted into thickest part reads 145°F, about 5 minutes per side. Brush the cut side of the bok choy with the reserved 2 tablespoons marinade. Grill the bok choy cut-side down until lightly charred, about 5 minutes.

Sprinkle the pork and bok choy with the cilantro before serving.

GROSS CARBS: **9 G**
NET CARBS: **9 G**

Braised Pork Chops with Fennel

These pork chops are simmered in a flavorful sauce that features vermouth, a botanically flavored wine that's featured in classic cocktails like a Negroni.

1 fennel bulb, stalks removed
2 teaspoons salt, plus more as needed
½ teaspoon pepper, plus more as needed
¾ teaspoon hot paprika
Three 1-inch-thick bone-in pork chops
2 tablespoons olive oil
½ yellow onion, thinly sliced
2 garlic cloves, thinly sliced
1 teaspoon minced fresh thyme
½ cup low-sodium chicken broth
½ cup dry vermouth
1 teaspoon Dijon mustard
½ teaspoon finely grated lemon zest
1 teaspoon fresh lemon juice

Trim the top and bottom off the fennel bulb and cut it in half. Cut each half lengthwise into ¼-inch-thick slices.

In a small bowl, combine the salt and pepper and ½ teaspoon of the paprika. Sprinkle both sides of the pork chops with the paprika mixture.

In a large lidded skillet or sauté pan over medium-high heat, heat the olive oil until shimmering. Add the pork chops and sear until golden brown on both sides, 6 to 7 minutes total. Transfer to a plate and set aside.

Reduce the heat to medium and add the fennel, onion, garlic, thyme, and the remaining ¼ teaspoon paprika to pan. Season with salt and pepper. Sauté until the fennel begins to brown, about 5 minutes. Add the broth and vermouth and bring to a boil, scraping up any browned bits from the bottom of the pan. Return the pork chops and any accumulated juices on the plate to pan. Cover, reduce the heat to low, and simmer until the chops are firm and they read 140°F inside, 8 to 10 minutes. Remove the pork chops to a clean plate, tent with foil, and let rest.

Increase the heat to medium and simmer the sauce, uncovered, until reduced by about one-third and slightly thickened, about 3 minutes. Remove from the heat, add the Dijon mustard, lemon zest, and lemon juice. Season with salt and pepper and serve over the pork chops.

GROSS CARBS: **13.5 G**
NET CARBS: **10.5 G**

Pork Loin with Rosemary and Dijon Mustard

SERVES 8

When trying to eat healthfully, pork tenderloin is a fabulous choice of protein. It's typically very lean and easy to prepare. This recipe combines pork with two classic flavors: fresh rosemary and spicy Dijon mustard.

One 4-pound boneless pork loin
2 tablespoons Dijon mustard
2 tablespoons chopped red onion
2 teaspoons salt
½ teaspoon pepper
1 garlic clove, minced
2 tablespoons chopped fresh rosemary

Preheat the oven to 350°F.

Trim any excess fat from the pork loin, leaving a thin layer of fat over the top. Evenly rub the pork loin with the Dijon mustard, followed by the onion, salt, pepper, and garlic. Sprinkle the rosemary over the top.

Place the pork on a rack in a roasting pan and roast for 20 minutes. Reduce the oven temperature to 300°F and continue roasting for about 1 hour more, or until a meat thermometer inserted into the thickest part of the pork loin reads 145°F. Transfer the pork to a cutting board, tent with foil, and let rest for 10 minutes before slicing.

GROSS CARBS: **0.5 G**
NET CARBS: **0.5 G**

Slow Cooker Roast Pork Shoulder with German Spices

SERVES 8

Pork shoulder is the perfect meat to cook in a slow cooker—the extended cooking time makes the meat incredibly tender. Arrowroot is a natural thickener used instead of flour in some recipes.

1 tablespoon caraway seed
1½ teaspoon dried marjoram
1 teaspoon salt
½ teaspoon pepper
3 pounds boneless pork shoulder
1 tablespoon olive oil
½ cup water
2 tablespoons white wine vinegar
8 ounces low-fat sour cream
4 teaspoons arrowroot

In a small bowl, combine the caraway seed, marjoram, salt, and pepper. Sprinkle the mixture over the pork shoulder and rub it into the roast with your fingers.

In a large skillet or sauté pan over medium-high heat, heat the olive oil until shimmery. Brown the meat on all sides, drain off the fat, and place the meat in a slow cooker.

Add the water to the pan, bring to a boil, and stir to loosen any browned bits from the bottom of the pan. Pour the pan juices and the vinegar into the cooker. Cover the cooker and cook on low for 7 hours or high for 3½ to 4½ hours. Remove the pork from the cooker and tent with foil to keep warm.

Skim any fat from the juices in the slow cooker, measure out 1¼ cup juices (add water if there's less than that amount), pour into a small saucepan, and bring to a boil.

In a medium bowl, combine the sour cream and arrowroot. Whisk the hot juices into the sour cream mixture, and return the mixture to the saucepan. Cook, stirring, over medium heat until the gravy is thickened. Slice the pork and serve with the gravy.

GROSS CARBS: **3 G**
NET CARBS: **2.5 G**

Beef Stir-Fry with Mushrooms and Swiss Chard

Stir-frying meat and vegetables is a quick way to get dinner on the table. By using thinly sliced ingredients and very high heat, you go from raw to done in 10 minutes. While this recipe calls for beef, substitute any other meat if you'd like.

1 pound boneless sirloin steak, cut into ¼-inch-thick slices
1 tablespoon plus 2 teaspoons cornstarch
1 tablespoon plus 2 teaspoons balsamic vinegar
4 teaspoons reduced-sodium soy sauce
2 teaspoons packed light brown sugar
⅓ cup water
3 tablespoons olive oil
3 garlic cloves, thinly sliced
½ red onion, cut into thin wedges
4 ounces white mushrooms, sliced
1 bunch Swiss chard, stems cut into ½-inch pieces, leaves shredded
Salt and pepper
Juice of ½ lemon

In a medium bowl, toss the beef with 1 tablespoon of the cornstarch, 1 tablespoon of the vinegar, and 2 teaspoons of the soy sauce.

In another medium bowl, stir the brown sugar, the remaining 2 teaspoons cornstarch, the remaining 2 teaspoons vinegar, the remaining 2 teaspoons soy sauce, and the water until dissolved.

In a large nonstick skillet or sauté pan over high heat, heat 1 tablespoon of the olive oil. Add the beef and cook, stirring occasionally, until just cooked through, 2 to 3 minutes. Transfer the beef to a bowl and wipe out the pan.

Heat the remaining 2 tablespoons olive oil in the pan over high heat. Add the garlic and onion and stir-fry for 2 minutes. Add the mushrooms and chard stems and stir-fry until tender, about 4 minutes. Season with salt and pepper. Add the chard leaves and stir-fry until wilted, about 1 minute. Give the brown sugar mixture a stir and add it to the pan along with the beef, stirring until thickened, about 1 minute. Add the lemon juice and season with salt and pepper.

GROSS CARBS: **13 G**
NET CARBS: **11 G**

Cheeseburger-Stuffed Peppers

SERVES 4

Simple green bell peppers are the perfect vessel for meat, veggies, and cheese. This version is topped with Cheddar, giving it an all-American flavor. Once the stuffed peppers are assembled, you can freeze them to bake later.

2 green bell peppers, halved lengthwise and seeded
1 pound ground beef
¼ cup chopped onion
1 garlic clove, minced
½ cup chopped tomato
Salt and pepper
6 ounces Cheddar cheese, shredded

Preheat the oven to 350°F.

In a large saucepan over high heat, bring 3 cups water to a boil. Add the bell peppers and boil for 3 minutes; drain and set aside.

In the same saucepan, brown the ground beef, onion, and garlic for 6 to 8 minutes. Drain off the fat and stir in the tomato. Season with salt and pepper. Reduce the heat to medium-high. Cook until the tomatoes are hot and then stir in 4 ounces of the Cheddar cheese.

Put the pepper halves in an 8-inch square baking pan and fill each half with the beef mixture. Sprinkle the remaining 2 ounces Cheddar over the top and bake for 20 to 25 minutes.

GROSS CARBS: **9.5 G**
NET CARBS: **8 G**

Stuffed Cabbage Rolls

This dish is believed to have originated in Europe, where cabbage leaves would be wrapped around a mixture of meat, spices, and grains. Fillings and sauces vary widely depending on the region, but all are delicious. The one that follows is a classic rendition, minus the grains.

Tomato Sauce
2 tablespoons olive oil
1 cup chopped onion
2 teaspoons minced garlic
One 28-ounce can peeled tomatoes with juice
1 cup canned tomato sauce
2 tablespoons packed light brown sugar
Salt and pepper

1 head green cabbage

Ground Beef Filling
1¼ pounds ground beef
½ cup minced onion
1 teaspoon minced garlic
2 eggs, lightly beaten
2 tablespoons ketchup
1 tablespoon dried dill
½ teaspoon salt
¼ teaspoon pepper

To prepare the tomato sauce: In a medium lidded saucepan over medium heat, heat the olive oil and sauté the onion and garlic until soft and lightly browned, about 3 minutes. Break up the tomatoes with your hands and add to the pan with their juice, and then add the canned tomato sauce and brown sugar. Season with salt and pepper. Reduce the heat to low, cover, and simmer gently for 45 minutes.

Preheat the oven to 400°F.

Bring a large pot of salted water to a boil over high heat. Cut the core from the cabbage and place the entire cabbage head into the water. As the leaves become softened, remove them one by one and place in a colander.

To prepare the ground beef filling: In a large bowl, add the ground beef, onion, garlic, eggs, ketchup, dill, and salt and pepper, and mix well with your hands.

Take a large cabbage leaf and carefully cut out the stiff rib at the base. Place $\frac{1}{3}$ cup filling near the stem end of the leaf. Fold the sides of the leaf over the filling and roll up. Transfer, seam-side down, to a large baking dish and repeat with the other leaves until all the filling is used up.

Pour the tomato sauce over the cabbage rolls, cover tightly with foil, and bake for about 45 minutes or until a thermometer reads 180°F when inserted into a cabbage roll.

GROSS CARBS: **18 G**
NET CARBS: **15 G**

Skirt Steak with Garlic-Herb Sauce

SERVES 6

Skirt steak can be a bit tough, so it's best either cooked very slowly or, as in this recipe, seared quickly over high heat. When cutting this piece of beef, make sure to cut across the grain to make it as tender as possible.

Garlic-Herb Sauce
1 garlic clove, minced
½ teaspoon salt
1 cup chopped fresh cilantro
¼ cup olive oil
2 tablespoons fresh lemon juice
⅛ teaspoon cayenne pepper

1 teaspoon ground cumin
½ teaspoon salt
½ teaspoon black pepper
One 2-pound skirt steak, cut crosswise into 3- to 4-inch pieces

To make the garlic-herb sauce: Place the garlic and salt in a small bowl. Place the garlic and salt and in a small bowl and mash to a paste. Transfer to a blender and add the cilantro, olive oil, lemon juice, and cayenne, then blend until smooth.

In a small bowl, combine the cumin, salt, and pepper. Pat the steak dry, then rub both sides with the cumin mixture.

Heat an oiled well-seasoned grill pan, skillet, or sauté pan over high heat until hot but not smoking. Grill the steak in two batches, turning occasionally, for about 2 minutes per batch for thin pieces or 6 to 8 minutes per batch for thicker pieces. Drizzle the steak with the garlic-herb sauce before serving.

GROSS CARBS: **1 G**
NET CARBS: **1 G**

Rib-Eye Steaks with Blue Cheese

Red meat and rich blue cheese are a natural pairing—the saltiness of the cheese cuts through the richness of the beef. Use Roquefort, Gorgonzola, or classic blue cheese, and you'll be guaranteed a delicious dish.

¼ cup butter, at room temperature
¼ cup crumbled blue cheese
3 tablespoons chopped toasted walnuts
Salt and pepper
1 tablespoon olive oil
Four ¾-inch-thick rib-eye steaks

In a medium bowl, combine the butter and blue cheese. Stir in the walnuts. Season with salt and pepper.

In a large heavy skillet or sauté pan over medium-high heat, heat the olive oil. Sprinkle both sides of the steaks with salt and pepper and sauté until brown and cooked to desired doneness, about 4 minutes per side for medium-rare. Transfer the steaks to plates and top each with 1 heaped tablespoon of the blue cheese–walnut butter.

GROSS CARBS: **1 G**
NET CARBS: **0.5 G**

Poultry, Pork, and Beef

Desserts

Grapefruit and Mint Sorbet

Cherry Sorbet

Mascarpone with Fresh Fruit

Strawberry and
Pomegranate Mousse

Spiced Pears

Grilled Peaches with Brown Sugar
and White Chocolate

Frozen Bananas with Chocolate
and Coconut

Gingerbread Crisps

Almond and Raspberry Jam
Thumbprint Cookies

Peanut Butter Cookies with
Sea Salt

Chocolate Chip Cookies

Popcorn Balls with Everything

Chocolate Bark with Nuts

Chocolate Truffles

Almond Cheesecake Bars

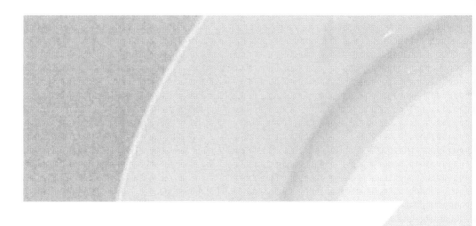

CHAPTER FOURTEEN

Desserts

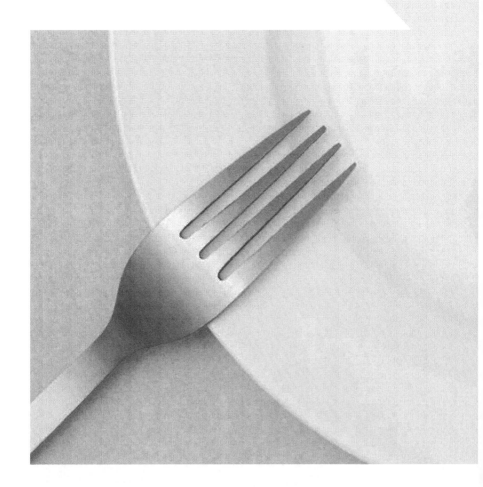

Grapefruit and Mint Sorbet

This tart sorbet is the perfect dessert for a hot day. The vodka helps give it a nice slushy consistency since vodka doesn't freeze. You can store the sorbet for up to 1 week in an airtight container in the freezer.

1 heaped tablespoon freshly grated grapefruit zest
3¾ cups pink grapefruit juice (not from concentrate)
¼ cup liquid honey
3 tablespoons cranberry juice concentrate
1½ tablespoons vodka
10 fresh mint leaves plus 2 teaspoons finely chopped fresh mint

Put a quart-size or larger container in the freezer to chill.

In a large saucepan over medium-high heat, combine the grapefruit zest, grapefruit juice, honey, cranberry juice concentrate, and vodka. Bring to a simmer and stir until the honey dissolves. Stir in the whole mint leaves.

Remove from the heat and set aside for 1 hour for the flavors to deepen.

Using a fine-mesh sieve or colander lined with cheesecloth, strain the mixture into a medium bowl, extracting as much liquid as possible. Stir in the chopped mint. Cover and refrigerate 3 hours or up to 3 days.

Process the mixture in an ice-cream maker according to the manufacturer's instructions for about 30 minutes. Transfer the sorbet to the chilled container and freeze until firm, about 2 hours.

GROSS CARBS: **19 G**
NET CARBS: **19 G**

Cherry Sorbet

Delicious cherries are the star of this dessert. You can use sweet cherries or sour cherries, and if they aren't in season, frozen cherries are just as good. If you go with sour cherries, you may need a little more confectioner's sugar.

4 cups pitted cherries
1 cup water
3 tablespoons confectioner's sugar

In a blender, purée the cherries, water, and sugar. Strain through a fine-mesh sieve, pressing on the solids to extract as much liquid as possible. Discard the solids and process the liquid in an ice-cream maker according to the manufacturer's instructions until slushy. Transfer to an airtight container and freeze until ready to serve.

If you don't have an ice-cream maker, pour the strained mixture into a 9-by-13-inch baking pan and place the pan on a level surface in the freezer. Freeze, scraping with a fork every 30 minutes and moving the frozen edges in toward the center, until firm and slushy, about 3 hours.

GROSS CARBS: **11 G**
NET CARBS: **10 G**

Mascarpone with Fresh Fruit

Mascarpone is a creamy Italian cheese used in all kinds of desserts like tiramisu. In this dessert, the cheese and fruit are served in cups of phyllo dough, which can typically be found in the frozen-food aisle of the supermarket. It can be a little challenging to work with, so don't get frustrated if at first you have to throw out a few sheets of phyllo.

3 sheets phyllo dough
¼ cup mascarpone cheese
¼ cup finely chopped pineapple
¼ cup nonfat raspberry yogurt
Small block of chocolate, for garnish

Preheat the oven to 350°F.

Layer the phyllo sheets on top of each other. Using a 2½- to 3-inch cookie cutter, cut out 12 rounds and press them into the cups of mini muffin tins. Bake until golden brown and crisp, about 7 minutes. Let cool.

In a small bowl, combine the mascarpone, pineapple, and raspberry yogurt. Spoon the mascarpone mixture into the cooled phyllo cups. Using a vegetable peeler, shave some of the chocolate on top and serve.

GROSS CARBS: **13 G**
NET CARBS: **12.5 G**

Strawberry and Pomegranate Mousse

SERVES 4

If you've ever wondered how jellies and puddings get their consistency, the answer is unflavored gelatin. Available in packets in the baking aisle, it's also a great tool for home cooks who want to make dishes like this mousse.

2 cups fresh strawberries, or 10 ounces thawed frozen strawberries
⅛ teaspoon salt
1 envelope unflavored gelatin
½ cup pomegranate juice
¼ cup sugar
One 7-ounce container 2% plain Greek yogurt

In a food processor, purée the strawberries and salt.

In a small bowl, sprinkle gelatin over ¼ cup of the pomegranate juice. Let stand for a few minutes until the gelatin has softened.

In a small saucepan, combine the remaining ¼ cup pomegranate juice and the sugar. Bring to a simmer and stir in the softened gelatin. Cook over very low heat, stirring, until the gelatin and the sugar are fully dissolved, about 1 minute.

Add the gelatin mixture to the strawberry purée in the food processor and process until combined. Add the yogurt and process briefly to blend.

Spoon into four small bowls or glasses and cover. Refrigerate 2 hours or until chilled and set.

GROSS CARBS: **11 G**
NET CARBS: **10 G**

Spiced Pears

When the weather begins to cool, we often crave desserts that feature warm autumnal fruits, like this one with ripe pears, brown sugar, and spices. If you can, use Bosc pears because they are likelier to keep their shape.

3 ripe but firm pears, cored and cut into ¼-inch slices
1 tablespoon lemon juice
2 tablespoons unsalted butter
3 tablespoons packed light brown sugar
½ teaspoon ground cinnamon
½ teaspoon ground ginger
¼ teaspoon ground cloves
Pinch of salt

In a medium bowl, toss the pears with the lemon juice.

In a large deep lidded skillet or sauté pan over medium heat, melt the butter. Stir in the pears. Reduce the heat to medium-low, cover, and cook, stirring once halfway through, for 10 minutes.

In a small bowl, combine the brown sugar, cinnamon, ginger, cloves, and salt. Add the sugar mixture to the pan with the cooked pears. Increase the heat to medium and cook, stirring often, until the pears are tender and glazed, 4 to 6 minutes. Serve warm.

GROSS CARBS: **20 G**
NET CARBS: **17 G**

Desserts

Grilled Peaches with Brown Sugar and White Chocolate

SERVES 8

When it's hot outside, why turn the oven on just to make dessert? Keep the grill going after making burgers and you can quickly create a delicious, healthful dessert.

4 tablespoons butter, melted
2 tablespoons packed light brown sugar
½ teaspoon ground cinnamon
4 peaches, halved and pitted
⅓ cup chopped white baking chocolate
3 tablespoons chopped pecans

Lightly coat a grill rack with oil or cooking spray. Preheat the grill to medium.

In a small bowl, combine the butter, brown sugar, and cinnamon. Add the peaches, one half at a time, toss to coat, and place on a plate. After you've coated all the peach halves, set aside the remaining butter mixture for later.

Place the peaches cut-side down on the grill and cook for 5 minutes.

Turn all the peaches over and fill the cavities with the white chocolate, dividing it equally among the 8 halves. Drizzle with the remaining butter mixture. Cover and grill for 4 to 5 minutes more or until the peaches are tender and begin to caramelize. Sprinkle with the pecans and serve.

GROSS CARBS: **14 G**
NET CARBS: **13 G**

Frozen Bananas with Chocolate and Coconut

SERVES 12

With only three ingredients, this might be the easiest dessert ever. Melt the chocolate in the microwave on medium—just make sure to check on it and give it a good stir every 20 seconds. If you don't like coconut, substitute pecans.

4 large ripe bananas, peeled and cut crosswise into thirds
¾ cup semisweet chocolate chips, melted
¼ cup unsweetened shredded coconut

Line a baking sheet with parchment paper.

Insert a Popsicle stick into each piece of banana. Coat each piece with the melted chocolate, using a rubber spatula, and sprinkle with the coconut before the chocolate begins to harden.

Place the bananas on the baking sheet and freeze, about 2 hours.

GROSS CARBS: **6 G**
NET CARBS: **4 G**

Desserts

Gingerbread Crisps

MAKES 15

These cookies have all the flavors of gingerbread men but are much thinner, so they carry far fewer carbs. The crystallized ginger adds a sharp, spicy punch.

Cooking spray for baking sheets
¾ cup whole-wheat pastry flour
½ teaspoon baking powder
½ teaspoon ground cinnamon
½ teaspoon ground ginger
¼ teaspoon salt
⅛ teaspoon baking soda
Pinch of ground cloves
⅓ cup packed light brown sugar
2 tablespoons melted unsalted butter
2 tablespoons molasses
1 tablespoon milk
1 egg, separated
2 tablespoons finely chopped crystallized ginger

Preheat the oven to 350°F. Line three rimmed baking sheets with parchment paper and lightly coat with cooking spray.

In a small bowl, sift together the flour, baking powder, cinnamon, ginger, salt, baking soda, and cloves.

In the bowl of a stand mixer fitted with a paddle attachment, combine the brown sugar, butter, molasses, milk, and egg yolk. Beat on medium-high speed until smooth, about 1 minute. Add the flour mixture and mix on low, increasing the speed gradually to medium-high, until a ball of dough forms, about 3 minutes.

Lightly coat two new pieces of parchment paper with cooking spray. Sandwich the dough between the parchment (with the sprayed sides touching the dough) and, using a rolling pin, roll out the dough until it is very thin, about 1/16 inch thick. Freeze for 30 minutes to allow the dough to get really firm. Cut out the cookies with 2-inch round cookie cutters and transfer them to the prepared baking sheets.

In a small bowl, whisk the egg white. Brush the tops of the cookies with the egg white. Sprinkle with the crystallized ginger.

Bake until golden, rotating the sheets about halfway through, 10 to 12 minutes total. Let cool for a few minutes on the sheets and then transfer to a rack to cool.

GROSS CARBS: **12 G**
NET CARBS: **12 G**

Almond and Raspberry Jam Thumbprint Cookies

MAKES 48

Thumbprint cookies are a classic dessert. The holes can be filled with anything from hazelnut spread to jam. This is also a great recipe to make with kids—let them help you press the indentations into the cookie dough balls.

1½ cups blanched slivered almonds
1 cup (2 sticks) butter, at room temperature
¾ cup sugar
½ teaspoon almond extract
2 cups all-purpose flour
⅛ teaspoon salt
¼ cup seedless sugar-free raspberry jam

Preheat the oven to 350°F. Line two baking sheets with parchment paper.

Place the almonds on a baking sheet and toast for 5 minutes or until golden. Let cool. Pulse in a food processor until finely chopped.

In a large mixing bowl, with an electric mixer, beat the butter, sugar, and almond extract at medium speed until light and fluffy. Beat in the chopped almonds. Reduce the speed to low and beat in the flour and salt until just combined.

Shape the cookie dough into 1-inch balls. Place the balls 2 inches apart on the prepared baking sheets. Press your index finger into the center of each ball to make a well. Bake for 6 minutes.

Remove from the oven, carefully re-press each fingerprint, and spoon about ¼ teaspoon of the jam into each. Bake for 6 to 8 minutes more or until the edges are golden. Let the cookies cool on a wire rack.

GROSS CARBS: **9 G**
NET CARBS: **9 G**

Peanut Butter Cookies with Sea Salt

Chocolate isn't the only flavor that benefits from a sprinkling of sea salt—peanut butter also shines. Let these cookies cool for a little bit in the pan before you put them on the cooling rack—they are a bit delicate when hot because they don't have any flour in them.

1 cup peanut butter
1 cup sugar
1 teaspoon pure vanilla extract
1 egg, lightly beaten
Coarse sea salt for sprinkling

Preheat the oven to 350°F. Line two rimmed baking sheets with parchment paper.

In a medium bowl, combine the peanut butter, sugar, vanilla, and egg. Spoon 1 tablespoon of the mixture onto a prepared baking sheet. Repeat until baking sheets are filled with cookies spaced 1½ inches apart. Using the tines of a fork, flatten the balls twice to make a crisscross pattern on top. Sprinkle with sea salt.

Bake until golden around the edges, about 10 minutes, switching placement of baking sheets halfway through. Let cool on the pans for a few minutes before transferring the cookies to racks to cool.

GROSS CARBS: **14 G**
NET CARBS: **13 G**

Chocolate Chip Cookies

When it comes to desserts, it doesn't get much better than chocolate chip cookies. If you forgot to set out the butter to soften in advance, just cut it up into smaller chunks and let them sit out on a plate.

½ cup instant oats
½ cup whole-wheat pastry flour
½ teaspoon baking powder
¼ teaspoon baking soda
½ teaspoon salt
⅓ cup packed light brown sugar
¼ cup honey
3 tablespoons unsalted butter, at room temperature
3 tablespoons canola oil
1¼ teaspoons pure vanilla extract
1 egg
¾ cup pecans, coarsely chopped
1 cup bittersweet chocolate chips

In a food processor or blender, process the oats until they resemble a fine powder.

In a medium bowl, whisk together the oats, flour, baking powder, baking soda, and salt.

In a large bowl, using an electric mixer, beat the brown sugar, honey, butter, oil, and vanilla until well combined. Beat in the egg. Add the oats mixture and beat on low speed until combined. Stir in the pecans and chocolate chips. Refrigerate the dough for 1 hour or up to overnight.

Preheat the oven to 375°F. Line a baking sheet with parchment paper.

Drop level tablespoons of dough onto the baking sheet at least 2 inches apart (8 cookies should fit on a baking sheet). Bake until golden, 7 to 9 minutes. Cool on the baking sheet for 5 minutes before removing to a wire rack to cool. Repeat with the remaining dough. Store these cookies in an airtight container for up to 2 days.

GROSS CARBS: **12 G**
NET CARBS: **10 G**

Popcorn Balls
with Everything

Whether you're craving something salty or sweet, these delicious popcorn balls will be perfect. The mix of chocolate, pretzels, peanut butter, and cherries make for an irresistible treat. Individually wrap each ball in plastic wrap before storing so they don't stick together.

¼ cup agave nectar

¼ cup creamy peanut butter, at room temperature

6 heaped cups popped popcorn

2 tablespoons finely chopped dark chocolate-covered pretzels

2 tablespoons finely chopped dried cherries

Line two baking sheets with parchment paper.

In a small saucepan over medium heat, combine the agave nectar and peanut butter. Stir constantly until mixture begins to bubble, then cook for 15 seconds more, stirring continuously.

Pour the popcorn into a large bowl, and pour the peanut butter mixture over it. Mix with a wooden spoon until the popcorn is coated. Gently stir in the chocolate-covered pretzels and the cherries.

Dip your hands into a medium bowl filled with ice water and quickly press the popcorn mixture into 2-inch balls (each will be a heaped ¼ cup of the mixture). Lightly squeeze the balls to compress them. Place the balls on the prepared baking sheets. Let cool completely before wrapping each ball in plastic wrap and storing in an airtight container for up to 2 days.

GROSS CARBS: **13 G**
NET CARBS: **12 G**

Chocolate Bark with Nuts

Mix and match different chocolates and nuts to find your perfect bark. Dark chocolate and almonds go especially well together, plus you get antioxidants from the dark chocolate. Melt the chocolate in the top of a double boiler, stirring constantly.

2 cups semisweet, bittersweet, or milk chocolate chips, melted
1½ cups assorted nuts (hazelnuts, almonds, cashews), plus more
    finely chopped for sprinkling (optional)

Line a rimmed baking sheet with foil (take care to avoid wrinkles).

In a medium bowl, combine the melted chocolate and the nuts. With a rubber spatula, scrape the mixture onto the baking sheet and spread it into a rectangle approximately 12 by 9 inches. Sprinkle with finely chopped nuts, if desired. Refrigerate until set, about 20 minutes.

Transfer the bark and foil to a cutting board. Using a large sharp knife, cut the bark into 1½-inch-square pieces.

GROSS CARBS: **7 G**
NET CARBS: **6 G**

Chocolate Truffles

The key to making these truffles is to keep the mixture very cold. When rolling the balls, work quickly so your hands don't melt the chocolate.

⅔ cup heavy cream
¼ cup butter, at room temperature
1¼ cups semisweet chocolate chips
½ teaspoon pure vanilla extract
½ cup unsweetened cocoa

In a small saucepan over medium heat, heat the cream until it begins to simmer. Stir in the butter and cook until melted. Remove from the heat and stir in the chocolate chips and then the vanilla. Keep stirring until all the chocolate is melted. Let stand for 5 minutes. Whisk a few times with a wire whisk until the mixture is smooth and then transfer to a medium bowl. Chill until firm in the refrigerator, at least 4 hours.

Place the cocoa in a medium bowl. Using a small spoon, scoop out heaped teaspoonfuls of the truffle mixture. Roll it between the palms of your hands into 1-inch balls, then roll the balls in the cocoa to coat.

GROSS CARBS: **4 G**
NET CARBS: **4 G**

Almond Cheesecake Bars

MAKES 36

The three layers of these bars work together to create one perfect dessert. The crunchy, buttery crust complements the creamy cheesecake and light frosting.

Cooking spray for the baking sheet
2 cups all-purpose flour
1¼ cup butter, at room temperature
2 cups confectioner's sugar
8 ounces cream cheese, at room temperature
½ cup granulated sugar
2 teaspoons almond extract
2 eggs, lightly beaten
4 teaspoons milk

Preheat the oven to 350°F. Coat a 13-by-9-inch baking sheet with cooking spray.

Combine the flour, 1 cup of the butter, and ½ cup of the confectioner's sugar. Press the mixture into the bottom of the prepared baking pan. Bake until golden brown, 20 to 25 minutes.

In a small bowl, using an electric mixer, beat the cream cheese, granulated sugar, and 1 teaspoon of the almond extract until smooth. Add the eggs and beat on low until just combined. Pour the cream cheese mixture over the crust. Bake until the center is almost set, 15 to 20 minutes. Let the sheet cool on a wire rack.

In a small bowl, combine the remaining 1½ cups confectioner's sugar, the remaining ¼ cup butter, the remaining 1 teaspoon almond extract, and the milk and mix until smooth. Spread the frosting over the cooled layered cheesecake in the pan and refrigerate until chilled. Cut into bars. Store in the refrigerator.

GROSS CARBS: **15 G**
NET CARBS: **15 G**

Index

Index

Index

Index

Index

193

194

Index

31532262R00116

Printed in Great Britain
by Amazon